AN EVALUATION OF A CANCER INFORMATION TELEPHONE FACILITY

AN EVALUATION OF A CANCER INFORMATION TELEPHONE FACILITY

Can-Dial

Gregg S. Wilkinson, Ph.D.
Edwin A. Mirand, Ph.D., D.Sc.
Saxon Graham, Ph.D.

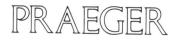

PRAEGER SPECIAL STUDIES • PRAEGER SCIENTIFIC

New York • Philadelphia • Eastbourne, UK
Toronto • Hong Kong • Tokyo • Sydney

Library of Congress Cataloging in Publication Data
Wilkinson, Gregg S.
   An evaluation of a cancer information telephone
facility, Can-Dial.

   Includes index.
   1. Cancer—Information services—New York (State)—
Buffalo. 2. Health education—New York (State)—
Buffalo. 3. Telephone in medicine.   4. Roswell Park
Memorial Institute. I. Mirand, Edwin A., 1926—
II. Graham, Saxon. III. Title.   [DNLM: 1. Health
Education—methods. 2. Information Services—
utilization. 3. Neoplasms. 4. Telephone—utilization.
QZ 200 W685e]
RC262.W55 1985   362.1'96994   84-26399
ISBN 0-03-000932-4 (alk. paper)

Published in 1985 by Praeger Publishers
CBS Educational and Professional Publishing, a Division of CBS Inc.
521 Fifth Avenue, New York, NY 10175 USA

56789 052 987654321

Printed in the United States of America on acid-free paper

INTERNATIONAL OFFICES

Orders from outside the United States should be sent to the appropriate address listed below. Orders
from areas not listed below should be placed through CBS International Publishing, 383 Madison Ave.,
New York, NY 10175 USA

Australia, New Zealand
Holt Saunders, Pty. Ltd., 9 Waltham St., Artarmon, N.S.W. 2064, Sydney, Australia

Canada
Holt, Rinehart & Winston of Canada, 55 Horner Ave., Toronto, Ontario, Canada M8Z 4X6

Europe, the Middle East, & Africa
Holt Saunders, Ltd., 1 St. Anne's Road, Eastbourne, East Sussex, England BN21 3UN

Japan
Holt Saunders, Ltd., Ichibancho Central Building, 22-1 Ichibancho, 3rd Floor, Chiyodaku, Tokyo, Japan

Hong Kong, Southeast Asia
Holt Saunders Asia, Ltd., 10 Fl, Intercontinental Plaza, 94 Granville Road, Tsim Sha Tsui East,
Kowloon, Hong Kong

**Manuscript submissions should be sent to the Editorial Director, Praeger Publishers, 521 Fifth
Avenue, New York, NY 10175 USA**

ACKNOWLEDGMENTS

A number of acknowledgments are due. Penny Hausler served as stenographer to the Can-Dial project throughout its lifetime. Craig Johnson was an assistant investigator and was responsible for many of the administrative details including daily operations and publicity. Russell Sciandra completed the calculations for the cost-effectiveness analysis and continues to be involved with the existing Can-Dial operation. Alice Sloan and Helen Oldfield completed most of the interviews. The late Bud Dillon helped facilitate the data processing activity. John Wilson was responsible for tabulating population counts based on census data and for computing rates. Numerous others, too many to mention, also contributed to the project in various ways.

Versions of the analysis upon which this report is based have appeared in the <u>American Journal of Public Health</u>, <u>Public Health Reports</u>, <u>International Journal of Health Education</u>, <u>Health Education Monographs</u>, and <u>Social Science and Medicine</u>.

The research reported in this work was supported in part by Contract N01-CN-45073 from the National Cancer Institute.

CONTENTS

LIST OF TABLES

TABLE

TABLE

LIST OF FIGURES

1

THE CAN-DIAL SYSTEM

The telephone is recognized as an important means of communication between parties and, increasingly, as a method of distributing information. In recent years, the variety of telephone information services available to the general public has evolved from time and temperature reports to include elements as diverse as religious messages, counseling and referral services, reports for hobbyists and sportsmen, and health information (Bartlett et al. 1973; Hickey 1971; Meyer et al. 1970). Best known among the dial-access health information services is Tel-Med, offering prerecorded audiotape messages on a wide variety of health topics and sponsored in many parts of the United States by local medical societies.

As a comprehensive cancer center, Roswell Park Memorial Institute in Buffalo, N.Y. is concerned with increasing public knowledge and improving health behavior with regard to cancer. Many cancers can be prevented; for instance, it has been estimated that 30 percent of cancer mortality is attributable to tobacco alone (Doll and Peto 1981). The prognosis for some cancers, such as those of the uterine cervix, colon, and breast, is improved when they are detected early. However, both prevention and early detection require knowledge and action on the part of the layman. Also, there is increasing demand on the part of cancer patients and their families for more information about the management and course of their disease.

Having perceived that a dial-access information service might be an alternative to pamphlets and the mass media as an information source, Roswell Park initiated the Can-Dial service in 1973. However, it was noted that there were no reports in the literature regarding the effectiveness of any dial-access health information system. Several questions demanded answers before such a system could be

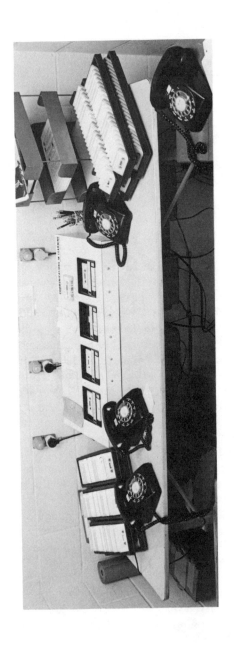

considered a significant contribution to cancer control: Does such an information system promote behavior leading to prevention and early detection of cancer? What population does it reach? What is the optimal method of operating and promoting the service? Does it demonstrate a high degree of client satisfaction? Such questions could be answered only by scientific evaluation of a pilot system.

A contract between Roswell Park and the National Cancer Institute was initiated in April 1974 to operate and evaluate the Can-Dial telephone cancer information service. Can-Dial was to make available to callers tape-recorded messages on cancer for sixteen hours a day and seven days a week.

Responsibilities of the staff were divided primarily between the operation and evaluation components of the system, with the entire project under the supervision of the principal investigator. During the course of the contract, two assistants to the principal investigator administered day-to-day operation, message preparation, and promotion of Can-Dial. The tape-playing system itself was operated by a crew of full- and part-time operators working in shifts, one to a shift. A stenographer provided secretarial services in both the operational and evaluative efforts.

The co-investigator, in consultation with the principal investigator and with the evaluation consultant, developed the evaluation instruments, supervised the collection of data, and analyzed the information gathered. Two interviewer/clerks conducted telephone interviews of 1,024 callers and 2,034 noncaller controls and tabulated statistics. A keypuncher/clerk transferred data to computer cards, and a part-time programmer assisted the co-investigator in analytical activities.

CAN-DIAL SYSTEM

The Can-Dial system consists of four telephones, each attached to an independent tape-playing machine. An individual wishing to use the system dials the advertised number and tells the operator who answers what taped message he or she wishes to hear. If the caller does not know which message is appropriate to answer the question, the operator can usually help select one. At this time the operator requests information from the caller as to name, address, etc., and completes the coded caller information sheet (see Appendix A). The operator then places the tape cassette bearing the selected message into the appropriate machine and hangs up the receiver, ready to take another call. An electronic signal at the end of each message shuts off the tape player and breaks the telephone connection.

Originally, Cousino tape players and tape cassettes were used. However, after two years the reliability of the players and, especially, the durability of the tapes were found to be less than expected. Therefore, a new, less expensive tape-playing system, designed especially for Can-Dial by Communications In Learning of Buffalo, was purchased. This machine operates on the same principle as the Cousino, but both the player and the tape cassettes are more compact. The reliability of both hardware and software was superior during the first year of its use, without any sacrifice of audio fidelity.

The messages were generally written by the public education staff and reviewed by appropriate members of the clinical staff. Messages were recorded in a sound studio to insure quality reproduction, an important consideration in telephone transmission. Cassette recordings were made from the master tape, which was retained in case replacement duplicates were needed. The Can-Dial library consisted of four copies of 51 tape messages, plus a set of Spanish translations of the first 28. Tapes were periodically reviewed and updated versions produced when necessary.

The volume of public use of Can-Dial is thought to have been related to the amount of publicity about it, which was achieved through distribution of pamphlets, printed advertisements, and short promotional spots via the electronic media.

PROMOTION

Approximately 910,500 pamphlets listing the topics and the telephone number were distributed. In addition to the standard "Cancer Facts" brochure, a series of pamphlets aimed at specific populations (blacks, rural dwellers, men, senior citizens) was developed. Brochures were distributed to the public in a variety of ways including: information racks in hospitals, clinics, libraries, and churches; through retail stores and pharmacies; through clubs and organizations to their members; through schools to students and parents; in employee paychecks; by direct residential mailing; through the American Cancer Society; and through other voluntary organizations and social service agencies.

Promotion through printed media consisted of several different modes. One of the most popular sources was a Can-Dial advertisement in the "White Pages" classified telephone directory. The White Pages Directory is published in the Buffalo, New York area in addition to the usual Telephone Directory with which most of us are familiar. Newspaper filler boxes were another frequently cited source. News releases about Can-Dial activities, especially the introduction of new messages, often led to articles that included the telephone number.

Public service announcements on television and radio were the third major type of promotion. For television, videotape announcements were prepared and distributed to stations. For radio, public service announcements dealing with the service in general and with specific tape topics were periodically prepared and distributed to stations. Licensed media are obliged by law to devote a specified amount of time to public service advertising, and Can-Dial seems to have received its fair share of such time. Unfortunately, many of these announcements were made late at night or early in the morning when the audience was small and Can-Dial was not operating.

While the electronic media certainly contribute to public awareness and use of Can-Dial, the printed media and pamphlets appear to be superior forms of advertising this service. To use Can-Dial, it is essential to know the phone number and helpful to know the topics available. In print this information is permanently available, while those learning it from electronic media must commit it to memory. Also, electronic media reach many people at the same instant, which can lead to heavy use of Can-Dial for a brief period. The printed media also reach a large number of people, but over a longer period of time, resulting in a more consistent level of use.

An analysis of the cost-effectiveness of the Can-Dial (Table 1.1) operation for the three years of operation (April 1974-April 1977) follows.* For purposes of this study, the costs of evaluation and related overhead were excluded from consideration, while costs of administration, operation, promotion, and related overhead were included.

Also excluded were contributed private costs, primarily those incurred by public service advertising (electronic and print) and by the American Cancer Society in its efforts to disseminate Can-Dial literature, as well as the costs incurred by various private and government agencies that distributed information to employees or clients. Any attempt to compute such contributed costs would be fragmentary at best.

The stress in this evaluation is on determining the costs incurred by this system, those likely to be incurred by similar systems, and the effect achieved. It is intended to serve as a practical indication as to whether a prerecorded telephone-access system can make a meaningful contribution to cancer control.

Costs for 1974 through 1977, totaling $120,782, were computed as seen in Table 1.1. In the three-year period Can-Dial received

------

*We are indebted to Russell Sciandra for his contributions to the analyses of cost-effectiveness.

Table 1.1 Cost of Operation, Exclusive of Evaluation

	Contract Supported	Roswell Park Supported	Total
Personnel (includes 25% overhead)			
Operators	$76,252		$76,252
Clerk-Typist (15%)	4,305		4,305
Administrator (15%)		$7,012	7,012
Assistant Administrator (15%)		4,037	4,037
Promotion	14,954		14,954
Equipment[a]	1,922		1,922
Telephone rental		2,916	2,916
Miscellaneous[b]	9,384		9,384
Total	$106,817	$13,965	$120,782

[a]Cost of new four line console and 216 cassettes. Costs of original Cousino tape players excluded ($4,300).

[b]Includes telephone installation, tape production, artwork, printing, and mailing of brochures, travel.

Note: Unless otherwise indicated, tables apply to the entire three-year period of Can-Dial's operation.

Source: Unless otherwise indicated, tables were compiled by the authors for this book.

77,571 local calls. Unit cost equals total cost divided by the volume of calls:

$$\frac{\$120,782}{77,571} = \$1.56 \text{ (unit cost)}$$

Unit costs could be reduced by increasing publicity and the resulting response. As can be seen from Table 1.1, publicity accounts for only 15 to 20 percent of costs.

Using assumptions drawn from analysis of data collected at the time of call and in follow-up interviews, some speculations regarding cost-effectiveness can be made. At the time of the call, 52.61 percent of callers giving their age were 20 or older. If those not giving their age were no different with respect to age from those who did, then 40,810 of Can-Dial's calls were made by adults. Since immediate benefits in terms of cancer control are more likely to be realized by educating adults than children, the cost of reaching adults is of particular interest:

$$\frac{\$120,782}{40,810} = \$2.96 \text{ (unit cost per adult call)}$$

In a follow-up survey of randomly selected callers, 39.8 percent reported taking some form of positive health-related action (modified smoking habit, visited a doctor, began breast self-examination, or reduced exposure to sun). After extrapolating these figures to the entire population of adult callers, we may assume that 16,038 callers took some action:

$$\frac{\$120,782}{16,038} = \$7.53 \text{ (unit cost per action)}$$

Of the callers surveyed, 11.7 percent reported seeing a physician or making an appointment to see a physician, while an additional 0.5 percent said they had a Pap test. An additional 4.5 percent reported that someone they talked to about the message went to a doctor or clinic. From this evidence we may speculate that 6,815 individuals visited a doctor:

$$\frac{\$120,782}{6,815} = \$17.72 \text{ (unit cost per doctor visit)}$$

Of course, such statistics are highly tentative. A complete discussion of Can-Dial's effects on callers may be found in the following chapters. It should be remembered that other, less tangible benefits may have been gained by callers. For instance, an additional 8.9 percent reported feeling more informed about cancer or having greater peace of mind after hearing the message.

Another way of expressing cost-effectiveness might be to say that the Can-Dial service was made available for three years to the people of Erie County at a cost of 10.9¢ per person:

$$\frac{\$120,782}{1,113,491} = \$0.1085$$
(population of
Erie County)

Even though the entire population did not use the system during its three years of existence, it was available to anyone at a very low cost.

2

METHODS OF EVALUATION

Evaluation was a major concern in the operation of the Can-Dial program. The system was conceived as an experiment with the evaluation comprising an integral component of the program. Evaluation activities were designed to: (1) provide immediate feedback that could be used for assessing progress, (2) provide information for more in-depth analyses, (3) ascertain differences between those who used the program and those who did not, and (4) ascertain the impact upon users, knowledge obtained, and motivation for using the program.

With this in mind, two means of collecting data were employed. The first entailed the monitoring of all calls received. At the time of the call, names and addresses were collected, as well as information regarding sex, age, occupation, topics selected, source of information, date of call, type of call, and phone number. This information allowed us to monitor who was using the program and to make needed changes upon becoming aware of certain groups that were not utilizing the system. For instance, it quickly became obvious to us that females used the program more than males, and that younger people called more frequently than the elderly. We were also able to monitor use of the program in various parts of Erie County by keeping track of census tract based upon address as well as township. Special efforts could then be made to increase advertising activities directed toward those groups and areas demonstrating low response. The data collected at the time of the call are primarily useful for that type of evaluation—often referred to as process evaluation. They also provided the basis for selecting our sample for subsequent telephone interviews.

The second method of evaluation entailed telephone interviews of a systematically selected sample of Can-Dial callers and a randomly selected sample of noncaller controls from the Erie County area. Noncallers were selected from the telephone directory. Information collected from callers included data pertaining to changes in behavior as a result of contact with the program, as well as motivations for using the system. Information collected from both callers and controls included data concerning education, marital history, occupation, contact with cancer patients, friends or relatives working in the health field, current health status, use of health services and orientation toward health, media use, and knowledge of cancer in terms of the seven warning signals. Identical interview schedules were used for both callers and noncaller controls, except that questions concerning action taken as a result of contact with the system and motivation for calling were included in the caller interview schedule only.

The manner in which data about calls were coded evolved by trial and error over a period of time. At first, information from callers was recorded on tape and later transcribed. It was then coded, keypunched, and put on computer tape. However, this method resulted in excessive handling of the data. Many data became lost because of unintelligible tapes and tape breakage. By having operators code this information at the time of the call, transcription and coding from transcripts were circumvented. Furthermore, data could then be keypunched the next day, after which they were immediately available for simple analyses via the countersorter. These data were then periodically put on computer tape for subsequent analysis.

We were interested in ascertaining patterns of use of the system as well as in knowing the basic characteristics of those who were using it. Through interviews, we hoped to discover the influence the program exerted upon the behavior of callers and the reasons why they called, as well as to explain differences in characteristics between callers and noncallers. We hypothesized that users of the program would be better educated, of higher socioeconomic status, more preventively oriented, and more concerned and aware of health matters than nonusers. We also hypothesized that experience with cancer or cancer-related health problems either in one's family, among friends, or experienced by individuals themselves would contribute to use of the program. Finally, we were interested in understanding differential use of media by callers and noncaller controls and communication patterns demonstrated by these groups.

QUALIFICATIONS

Several qualifications must be mentioned at this time. The first is that the Can-Dial program was viewed primarily as a public service.

Consequently, it was not necessary for callers to provide information in order to use the service. Individuals who did not wish to volunteer the information desired were still able to listen to the tapes they were interested in. This, of course, affects the data that we were able to collect since many individuals did not wish to give the information we requested. In such cases, operators attempted to obtain as much information as possible. Any errors that may be due to the withholding of information by certain groups of callers should in the long run be overcome because of the large numbers from whom information was received. Of course, we cannot guarantee that biases do not exist.

A second qualification concerns the necessity to limit the data gathered at the initial call. It would have been worthwhile to have asked individuals a number of questions contained in the call-back interviews. For instance, if knowledge of the seven danger signals had been determined at the time of the call and also during the call-back telephone interview several months afterward, we would have been able to examine knowledge as measured by these criteria both before and after contact with the program. This would have resulted in a pretest, post-test design. It would have allowed us to ascertain more confidently whether callers were actually retaining knowledge from contact with the program.

A third qualification concerns the validity of self-reports. Both the information obtained at the time of the call and that obtained through telephone interviews are based upon self-reports. It would have been desirable to have validated some of the responses, such as reports concerning physician visits or appointments with physicians or clinics. However, to do so would have required more resources than were available. There is a serious possibility that many of the respondents and their physicians would have viewed this as an invasion of privacy. Consequently, this type of validation was discarded.

The final qualification is that the sample of callers was based upon the names, addresses, and telephone numbers given by callers at the time of the call. Since not all individuals gave this information, the sample base, of necessity, is restricted. Furthermore, controls were selected through the telephone directory. It could be argued that not all individuals who have telephones are listed in the directory and that this could result in selection bias. However, most telephone users are listed; those who are not comprise a very small minority. Since this is a telephone information program, it would not have been of any value to contact indivividuals who do not have telephones at home, as they would be unlikely to contact the program in the first place.

In spite of these limitations, the data collected through the Can-Dial program served a useful purpose, providing us with an indication of the times that people utilized the system, the characteristics of those utilizing it, insight into reasons for using the program, and the influence of the program upon the users themselves.

3

CAN-DIAL RESPONSE

In this chapter we will be concerned with reporting results from the continuous monitoring of all calls received by the Can-Dial program. As was mentioned earlier, information was collected by the telephone operator at the time of contact with the program. This information, consisting of demographic characteristics as well as characteristics of the call itself, was coded by the operator at that time. These data were then keypunched within the next several days and entered onto magnetic computer tape for analysis.

TOTAL RESPONSE

By April 30, 1977, after slightly more than three years of operation, the Can-Dial program had received 108,282 calls. This included 77,571 calls from the Erie County area and 30,711 from outside the county. Since we were unable to include all of this information in our evaluation activities, and since it was necessary to set definite time frames, the materials contained in this report consist of data obtained only from the Erie County area from the beginning of April 1974 through the end of March 1977. During this time, information on 76,036 calls from the Erie County area was collected. This chapter will be devoted to reporting results of our evaluation efforts pertaining to patterns of response and the characteristics of callers.

MONTHLY RESPONSE

Throughout the three-year period, monthly response was consistent with respect to each month during the year. As demonstrated

Table 3.1 Monthly Response

| | Response | |
	Number	Percent
April	4,434	5.8
May	4,785	6.3
June	4,702	6.2
July	5,176	6.8
August	7,775	10.2
September	7,680	10.1
October	7,777	10.2
November	7,399	9.7
December	6,544	8.6
January	8,264	10.9
February	5,641	7.4
March	5,859	7.7
Total	76,036	99.9*

*Total differs from 100 percent due to rounding errors.

by Table 3.1, response was low during April, increased during May, June, and July, reached peaks during August, September, and October, remained high during November, December, and January, and then tended to decline during February and March. This was a consistent trend or pattern that we saw during each of the three years that Can-Dial was in operation. Although this pattern is somewhat difficult to explain, one possibility is that high response during the late summer and early September may be due in part to publication and distribution of the White Directory telephone classified pages. Many individuals, upon receiving their new White Directory, probably noticed the availability of the Can-Dial service and, out of curiosity or for other reasons, made a call. Interest in the program seemed to remain fairly high throughout the fall and early winter months, with the exception of January and the period around the holidays, when response fell each year. During the late winter and early spring, we always observed a decline in response that continued through the early summer. This decrease is understandable in light

of the beginning of the vacation season and the advent of more pleasur-
able weather in the Buffalo area. In any event, these monthly variations
in response were experienced in all three years of our operation.

DAILY RESPONSE

We were also interested in examining response for each day of
the week. Since we operated Can-Dial seven days a week, it is worthwhile to know the days on which response was highest for purposes of
cost control. As demonstrated in Table 3.2, greatest response was
experienced Monday through Thursday. Use tended to decline on Fri-
day and reached low points on Saturday and Sunday. An obvious impli-
cation is that programs such as Can-Dial can expect greatest use
during the five-day work week. If it is necessary, for reasons of
cost or otherwise, to restrict operation of such programs, periods
of greatest potential response will still be covered if weekend hours
are eliminated. However, it should be noted that 22 percent of all
calls were received during weekends.

Table 3.2 Daily Response

	Response	
	Number	Percent
Sunday	6,445	10.0
Monday	10,496	16.3
Tuesday	10,221	15.9
Wednesday	10,251	16.0
Thursday	10,040	15.6
Friday	9,261	14.4
Saturday	7,555	11.8
Total	64,269	100.0

HOURLY RESPONSE

Examination of hourly response is important since it allows us
to ascertain periods of the day during which maximum utilization of
the system occurred. Table 3.3 shows that the hours of greatest use
during the typical day were from 10 A.M. to 9 or 10 P.M. The two-

Table 3.3 Response by Hour

	Response	
	Number	Percent
8:00- 8:59 A.M.	1,423	2.6
9:00- 9:59 A.M.	2,699	4.9
10:00-10:59 A.M.	3,258	5.9
11:00-11:59 A.M.	3,489	6.3
12:00-12:59 P.M.	3,378	6.1
1:00- 1:59 P.M.	3,996	7.2
2:00- 2:59 P.M.	4,328	7.8
3:00- 3:59 P.M.	5,160	9.3
4:00- 4:59 P.M.	4,885	8.8
5:00- 5:59 P.M.	3,726	6.7
6:00- 6:59 P.M.	3,972	7.2
7:00- 7:59 P.M.	4,282	7.7
8:00- 8:59 P.M.	3,517	6.3
9:00- 9:59 P.M.	3,285	5.9
10:00-10:59 P.M.	2,461	4.4
11:00-11:59 P.M.	1,594	2.9
Total	55,453	100.0

hour periods from 8 to 9:59 A.M. and from 10 P.M. to midnight were the times of least response. Thus, if similar programs were operated from 10 in the morning until approximately 10 at night, times of greatest use would be covered. Operation of telephone information programs such as Can-Dial during a normal eight- or possibly twelve-hour work day will insure availability at those times when people are most likely to call.

SOURCE OF INFORMATION

Since the system was advertised by many different means, callers were asked where they heard about the Can-Dial program. Table 3.4 provides a listing of sources of information as reported by callers at the time of the call. The most frequently mentioned source of information was the White Directory telephone classified pages. General distribution of brochures and those distributed through schools constitute the second most frequent source of information. Finally, we find television and personal contact accounting for about 10 percent of the response, followed by the rest of the various sources.

Several implications are forthcoming. First, when all modes of distribution of pamphlets are grouped and considered, they account for about 36 percent of reported sources of information. However, it is necessary to keep in mind that this mode entails printing and some-times distribution costs. In contrast, other types of promotion entail

Table 3.4 Source of Information

	Response	
	Number	Percent
Television	5,578	10.0
Radio	1,776	3.2
Newspaper	3,104	5.6
Brochures	7,317	13.2
White Directory	16,443	29.6
Personal contact	5,199	9.3
School assignment	1,972	3.5
School distribution	7,972	14.3
Library	1,015	1.8
Doctor, dentist, hospital, or clinic	1,104	2.0
Brochure by mail	1,286	2.3
Bank, church, store, or community center	1,515	2.7
Other	1,361	2.5
Total	55,642	100.0

no cost since they involve public service time or space. Second, it is interesting to note that those modes that provided the telephone number and the topics in writing elicited greatest response. In fact, approximately 66 percent of the responses received implicated written sources of information. Programs of this type, in which there is a telephone number involved as well as a variety of topics that can be selected, probably require a certain amount of time for the individual to become aware of the number and of the possible topics from which a choice may be made. Other types of information sources such as the electronic media or personal contact also elicited some response, but at the same time they were less frequently cited than brochures and the White Directory. Brief radio or television announcements, although useful, were certainly less effective than written media.

TYPE OF CALL

Table 3.5 indicates the type of calls received by the Can-Dial program. New calls comprised approximately 62 percent of the response. About 18 percent were repeat calls, and approximately 7 percent were unknown. Other types of calls, including hang-ups and crank calls, comprised somewhere around 12 percent of the contacts.

Table 3.5 Response by Type of Call

| | Response | |
	Number	Percent
New call	41,724	62.3
Repeat call	12,256	18.3
Hang-up	4,406	6.6
Request for information	3,027	4.5
Wrong number	535	0.8
Unknown	4,976	7.4
Other	37	0.1
Total	66,961	100.2*

*Total differs from 100 percent due to rounding errors.

TOPICS OFFERED

Table 3.6 shows the topics offered according to their popularity. Topics were ranked according to the mean number of requests per month. From the beginning of the Can-Dial program, the most popular tapes were "If You Want to Give up Cigarettes" and "Cancer of the Breast." "The Effect of Cigarette Smoking on the Non-Smoker" as well as general tapes concerning cancer's warning signals and "What Is Cancer?" were also very popular. Media coverage of the relationship between radiation and thyroid cancer during several months of the Can-Dial operation resulted in considerable community interest in this subject. Subjects such as lung cancer, colo-rectal cancer, uterine cancer, cancer of the skin, leukemia, Hodgkin's disease, and the Pap test have also been popular. It is interesting that four of the thirteen most popular subjects concerned cigarette smoking. This may indicate public concern and a desire by many people either to give up smoking or to obtain more information and knowledge about it. The selection of topics showed that information pertaining to many known cancer problems and important sites was at least being distributed to the public.

DEMOGRAPHIC CHARACTERISTICS

Throughout its existence, the Can-Dial program experienced greater response from females than from males. Table 3.7 shows female exceeding male response by approximately a two to one margin. This relationship existed continuously throughout the program. We also experienced considerable age differences in response. If we examine the response rate per 10,000 of population for each 10-year age group as presented in Table 3.8, we note that response decreased from a high of 1,050/10,000 for the age interval 10 to 19 years of age to a low of 36.45/10,000 of population for those 70 and over (U.S. Department of Commerce, 1970). Thus, excluding those who are under 10 years of age, we find response decreasing in a steady fashion with increasing age. This relationship existed in spite of efforts to increase calls from the elderly. Promotional activities directed specifically toward retired people and their organizations were conducted without great success. This failure to reach the elderly prompted considerable concern since those 40 years of age and over are at increased risk for most forms of cancer. It may be that telephone information programs such as Can-Dial do not attract elderly individuals. Poor response may be a result of lack of interest, fear, denial, or a fatalistic outlook. Of course, we have no direct evidence of any of these and can only speculate as to possible reasons.

Table 3.6 Topics Selected

			Response	
	Date Issued	Number	Mean[a]	Rank[b]
If You Want to Give up Cigarettes	April 1974	9,772	271.4	1
Thyroid Cancer Following Radiation	January 1977	419	209.5	2
Cancer of the Breast	April 1974	4,663	129.5	3
Cancer's Warning Signals	April 1974	3,160	87.8	4
Effect of Cigarette Smoking on the Non-Smoker	April 1974	3,022	83.9	5
What Is Cancer?	April 1974	2,880	80.0	6
Lung Cancer	April 1974	2,383	66.2	7
Cancer of the Colon and Rectum	April 1974	2,345	65.1	8
Cancer of the Uterus	April 1974	2,258	62.7	9
Cancer of the Skin	April 1974	2,199	61.1	10
Leukemia	April 1974	1,927	53.5	11
Cigarette Smoking and the Pregnant Woman	April 1974	1,881	52.3	12
Questions and Answers about Smoking and Quitting	October 1974	1,489	51.3	13
Hodgkin's Disease	April 1974	1,834	50.9	14
What Is the Pap Test?	April 1974	1,823	50.6	15
Cancer Facts for the Teenager and Young Adult	October 1974	1,257	43.4	16
Cancer of the Brain	April 1974	1,535	42.6	17
Cancer of the Mouth	April 1974	1,495	41.5	18
Chemotherapy	April 1974	1,344	37.3	19
Cancer of the Stomach	April 1974	1,285	35.7	20
Breast Cancer Facts	October 1974	1,001	34.5	21
Cancer of the Bone	April 1974	1,208	33.6	22
Cancer of the Larynx	April 1974	1,186	32.9	23
Cancer of the Liver	August 1974	954	30.8	24
Cancer of the Prostate	April 1974	1,011	28.1	25
Cancer of the Bladder	August 1974	860	27.7	26

Topic	Date	[a]	[b]	
Questions and Answers about Smoking and Health	October 1974	731	25.2	27
Cigarette Smoking and Dental Problems	April 1974	826	22.9	28
Cancer of the Thyroid	April 1975	468	20.4	29
Cancer of the Pancreas	August 1974	588	19.0	30
What Is Roswell Park Memorial Institute?	April 1974	538	14.9	31
Radiation Therapy	April 1974	417	11.6	32
Words from a Hospital Chaplain	April 1974	402	11.2	33
Service and Rehabilitation Information	April 1974	354	9.8	34
The Economic Impact of Cancer on the Family	April 1975	135	5.9	35
Lymphomas and Multiple Myeloma	October 1975	64	3.8	36
Speech Therapy after Cancer Treatment	April 1975	69	3.0	37
Cancer Facts for the Senior Citizen	April 1975	67	2.9	38
Second Hand Smoke and Non-Smoker's Rights	October 1975	37	2.2	39
Air Pollution	October 1975	27	1.6	40
Cigarettes—The Economic Realities[c]	March 1977			
Childhood Cancers	March 1977			
Unproven Methods of Cancer Treatment—Risks and Dangers	March 1977			
Professional Assistance in Quitting Smoking	March 1977			
The Ex-Smoker's Guide to Staying Off Cigarettes	March 1977			
Smoking—The Beginning of a Habit	March 1977			
What Can Schools and Parents Do to Help Prevent Cigarette Smoking?	March 1977			
Important Information for School Teachers	March 1977			
Mammography—Is It for You?	March 1977			
Laetrile	March 1977			
Early Detection of Colon Cancer	March 1977			

[a]Monthly mean based upon calls received per months available.

[b]Rank order based upon monthly mean response

[c]Topics added late in March 1977

Wilkinson, Mirand, and Graham

Table 3.7 Response by Sex

| | Response | |
	Number	Percent
Male	23,295	36.1
Female	41,328	64.0
Total	64,623	100.1*

*Total differs from 100 percent due to rounding errors.

Other ways of reaching the elderly need to be developed and imple-
mented. Future endeavors need to be directed toward the aged if
cancer control efforts are to be successful in insuring that new modes
of control are applied to at-risk target populations (see also Wilkinson and Wilson 1983).

As may be seen from Table 3.9, response by occupation shows
the most frequent users to be students and housewives. Little vari-
ation is to be found among other occupational categories, although
the unemployed call almost as frequently as do professionals and
clerical workers. In all probability, the most insightful conclusion

Table 3.8 Response by Age

| Age | Response | | | |
	Number	Percent	Rate/10,000	Population
Under 10	1,341	2.6	66.98	200,204
10-19	22,908	44.9	1,050.27	218,116
20-29	11,240	22.0	755.27	148,821
30-39	6,356	12.5	545.86	116,440
40-49	4,638	9.1	327.48	141,627
50-59	3,150	6.2	248.09	126,971
60-69	1,154	2.3	131.85	87,527
70 and over	269	0.5	36.46	73,785
Total	51,056	100.1*	458.52	1,113,491

*Total differs from 100 percent due to rounding errors.

Table 3.9 Response by Occupation

	Response	
	Number	Percent
Professional or technical worker	2,125	5.1
Farmer or farm manager	13	0.0
Manager or official	495	1.2
Clerical or kindred worker	2,352	5.7
Sales worker	911	2.2
Craftsman or foreman	543	1.3
Operative or kindred worker	553	1.3
Private household worker	21	0.1
Service worker	1,223	3.0
Farm laborer or foreman	54	0.1
Laborer	1,095	2.6
Housewife	9,236	22.3
Student	20,496	49.4
Retiree	531	1.3
Self-employed worker	149	0.4
Unemployed worker	1,717	4.1
Total	41,514	100.1*

*Total differs from 100 percent due to rounding errors.

to be gleaned from these differences is that occupational groups that have more free time than others are more likely to utilize the Can-Dial program. For instance, students and housewives have access to telephones during major portions of the day, when Can-Dial was in operation. They are also likely to have the time in which to make calls as compared to other occupational groups. Of course, this is not to say that interest does not influence Can-Dial response from these groups. However, the much larger response by students and housewives, in all probability, results from more leisure time and access to the telephone.

Table 3.10 Response by Socioeconomic Quartile
          (per 10,000 population)

		Response		
Quartile	Number	Percent	Rate/10,000	Population
1 (High)	6,481	25.2	232.8	278,362
2	5,626	21.9	208.9	269,208
3	6,465	25.1	235.4	274,603
4 (Low)	7,167	27.8	255.4	280,621
Total	25,739	100.0	233.4	1,102,794

Socioeconomic status (SES) is of considerable interest to those
who are concerned with the utilization of health services and the adoption of health innovations (Ianni et al. 1960; Yeracaris 1961). It is
also useful for defining target populations. For instance, lower socioeconomic women are known to be at higher risk for such sites as
cervical cancer than are upper-class women. Several studies have
shown that, despite this, lower SES women are often among the lowest
users of Pap screening clinics (see Graham 1973). Also, lower SES
groups are often low utilizers of other types of health services.
Table 3.10 shows the distribution of Can-Dial response per 10,000
population for the Erie County area. For the county as a whole, quartile 4 demonstrates the best response, followed by quartiles 3 and 1.
The lowest response was received from quartile 2, which is upper
middle-class. We had originally hypothesized that response would
decrease with decreased socioeconomic status. The lower SES groups
are of particular interest since they comprise a segment of the population that is particularly in need of information regarding cancer
and various cancer control activities. These results show that this
information found its way to those who may have needed it the most.
However, these findings must be qualified since we have information
only on approximately one-third of the Can-Dial users. The other
two-thirds were individuals who were not asked such identifying information (18 or younger), or adults who refused to give their address
from which socioeconomic status could be computed. The response
rate was only 52 percent for those callers 20 and above. Even so,
these data provide some indication of the possible relevance of telephone information systems for dispensing health information to the
lower socioeconomic groups.
Table 3.11 provides an illustration of response per 10,000 by
town of residence, grouped into the central urban area, first-ring

Table 3.11 Response by Town of Residence

	Population	Frequency	Rate/10,000
Central Urban			
Buffalo	462,760	23,235	502.1
Lackawanna	28,657	1,164	406.2
First-Ring Suburbs			
Orchard Park	19,978	1,249	625.2
Lancaster	30,634	661	215.7
West Seneca	48,404	1,816	375.2
Cheektowaga	94,236	3,638	386.0
Hamburg/Blasdell	47,544	1,773	372.9
Kenmore/Tonawanda	129,180	1,877	145.3
Amherst/Williamsville	93,929	7,956	847.0
Depew	14,392	919	638.5
Rural			
Evans/Angola	14,570	1,336	916.9
Brant	2,672	66	247.0
Eden	7,644	309	404.2
North Collins/Collins	10,490	182	173.5
Concord/Springville	7,573	218	287.9
Sardinia	2,505	11	43.9
Holland	3,140	148	471.3
Colden	3,020	80	264.9
Boston	7,158	153	213.9
Aurora	14,426	531	368.1
Wales	2,617	69	263.7
Elma	10,011	333	332.6
Marilla	3,250	71	218.5
Alden	9,787	292	298.4
Akron/Newstead	6,338	168	265.1
Clarence	18,168	731	402.3
Grand Island	13,977	1,051	751.9

Table 3.12 Response by Socioeconomic Quartile and Residence
(per 10,000 population)

Quartile	Urban			Suburban			Rural			Total		
	Number	Rate/10,000	Population	Number	Rate/10,000	Population	Number	Rate/10,000	Population	Number	Rate/10,000	Population
1 (High)	4,180	268.0	155,980	2,632	242.2	108,659	891	227.9	39,101	7,703	276.7	303,740
2	2,871	260.5	110,224	2,273	204.2	111,338	954	219.7	43,419	6,098	226.5	264,981
3	3,031	268.7	112,785	2,802	235.2	119,121	802	194.4	41,247	6,635	241.6	273,153
4 (Low)	2,160	214.4	100,735	2,303	202.3	113,862	748	187.3	39,932	5,211	185.7	254,529
Total	12,242	255.2	479,724	10,010	212.5	452,980	3,395	207.4	163,699	25,647	232.6	1,096,403

suburbs, and rural townships. Overall response showed a tendency to decline from a high in the central urban area to somewhat lower among the first-ring suburbs, with lowest response being manifested by the rural exurbs. Although exceptions to this tendency were found, rural residents in Erie County comprised another group of low utilizers of the program.

This tendency is further documented when the rate of response per 10,000 of population is examined for SES quartile and residence. Note in Table 3.12 that the marginal rates for urban, suburban, and rural areas decrease as one moves from urban to rural place of residence. This tendency occurs consistently, with the exception of quartile 2. When the socioeconomic distribution of response within each geographic area is examined, we find little difference among urban callers between quartiles 1, 2, and 3. However, quartile 4 is considerably lower than the three higher quartiles. With respect to suburban callers, highest response came from quartiles 1 and 3, with lowest response being demonstrated by quartiles 2 and 4. Among rural callers, decreasing response is observed with decreasing socioeconomic status. These data indicate that response decreases with socioeconomic status when residence is taken into account. That is, as socioeconomic status decreases and as one moves from the central urban area to the rural exurbs, response also decreases. The decrease from urban to rural residence, however, is more consistent than is that from high to low socioeconomic status.

Table 3.13 illustrates the response by SES quartile and sex controlled for residence. Two important items are observed in this table. First, female response always exceeded male response for each quartile and for each area of residence. This finding seems to indicate that sex was a more important determinant of response to the Can-Dial program than socioeconomic status or residence. Second, the distribution within each sex grouping differs according to socioeconomic status for males when compared to females. Among urban dwellers, the highest rate of response for males occurred in quartile 1. On the other hand, the highest response for females (rate per 10,000 of population) occurred in quartile 3. For suburban and rural residents, the highest rate of response for both males and females occurred in quartile 1.

If we examine the lowest rates of response, we find that both males and females who lived in the city from quartile 4 demonstrated the lowest rate of response. The same holds true for suburban dwellers and for rural females. However, for males from rural areas, the lowest response was experienced from quartile 3, although the difference between quartiles 3 and 4 is very small. These data indicate the tendency for the highest response to be forthcoming from the upper whereas the lowest response tends to come from the lowest SES

Table 3.13 Response by Socioeconomic Quartile, Residence, and Sex (per 10,000 population)

Residence	Quartile	Response					
		Males			Females		
		Number	Rate/10,000	Population	Number	Rate/10,000	Population
Urban	1 (High)	1,522	212.5	71,635	2,549	302.2	84,345
	2	933	181.3	51,473	1,847	314.4	58,751
	3	973	183.4	53,050	1,969	329.6	59,735
	4 (Low)	745	157.1	47,407	1,341	251.5	53,328
Total		4,173	186.7	223,565	7,706	300.8	256,159
Suburban	1	868	165.5	52,422	1,680	298.7	56,237
	2	828	152.3	54,380	1,383	242.8	56,958
	3	927	161.5	57,405	1,793	290.5	61,716
	4	746	134.5	55,464	1,496	256.2	58,398
Total		3,369	153.4	219,671	6,352	272.3	233,309
Rural	1	313	162.0	19,317	558	282.0	19,784
	2	323	149.5	21,612	591	271.0	21,807
	3	269	131.9	20,388	514	246.4	20,859
	4	270	136.1	19,842	464	230.9	20,090
Total		1,175	144.8	81,159	2,127	257.7	82,540

Table 3.14 Reasons for Calling: First Reason Cited

	Response	
	Number	Percent
Desire to quit smoking	220	23.4
Curiosity	216	22.9
Desire for more knowledge	115	12.2
Interest in a specific topic	103	10.9
Current medical problem	94	10.0
Cancer in family	90	9.6
Possible cancer symptoms	45	4.8
Other illness in the family	22	2.3
Friend with cancer	22	2.3
Cancer patient	15	1.6
Total	942	100.0

Source: G. S. Wilkinson, E. A. Mirand, and S. Graham, Cancer Information by Telephone: A Two-Year Evaluation, Health Education Monographs, vol. 5, no. 3, pp. 251-65, 1977. Reprinted with permission of the Society for Public Health Education, Inc.

groups when residence is controlled. This tends to occur regardless of place of residence with few exceptions. Also, females display higher rates of response than do males.

A matter of considerable interest is the reason or reasons why individuals call the Can-Dial program. Table 3.14 presents a breakdown of the first reasons given by Can-Dial cases. By far the greatest majority cited the wish to quit smoking as a reason, followed by those who stated they were curious. Next most frequent were those individuals who wished to obtain more knowledge and those who had medical problems or were interested in specific types of cancer. Cancer in the family also comprised an important reason, followed by several other justifications. Interest in quitting smoking coincided with the popularity of smoking-related topics. This demonstrates that many were concerned about the possible relationship between cigarette smoking and lung cancer and wished to obtain more information about this problem. It also may indicate that many desired to cut down or quit smoking altogether. In all probability, the past educational campaigns offered by the American Cancer Society and other organizations had aroused the concern of many individuals. It is interesting to note that, if we group all those reasons concerning experience with cancer or medical problems, approximately 30 percent of respondents then fall into this category. Thus, a large portion of Can-Dial callers were those who had had direct experience with cancer or were currently experiencing some type of illness or medical problem.

In this chapter, we have been concerned with describing patterns of response and general characteristics of Can-Dial callers. We have noted various monthly, daily, and hourly variations in calls, our experience with regard to sources of information cited by callers, types of calls received, and the rank order of popular topics. We found that: females called more often than males; the young called more often than the elderly; there was some tendency for the lower SES groups to call less often than higher groups when residence was controlled; and there was a definite tendency for rural dwellers to call much less frequently than urban or suburban dwellers. Finally, we have noted that concern about smoking and experience with medical problems or cancer in the family comprised a large motivating factor for many individuals calling Can-Dial. In the next chapter, we shall be concerned with results of telephone interviews with a sample of Can-Dial callers and a randomly selected sample of noncaller controls.

4

COMPARISON OF CALLERS
AND NON-CALLER CONTROLS

The second method of evaluation employed entailed call-back telephone interviews of a systematically selected sample of Can-Dial callers and a randomly selected comparison sample of noncaller controls from the Erie County area. A total of 1,024 caller interviews and 2,034 control interviews were completed. Table 4.1 shows the completion rate of caller and control interviews experienced during the study.

Attempts were made to interview 1,459 callers and 2,809 noncaller controls. Seventy percent of the caller interviews were completed, and the refusal rate was 4.4 percent. About 24 percent of the caller contacts initiated were not completed because of wrong numbers, changes in address, changes in the telephone number, or death of the respondent. One percent of the interviews were not completed because of illness or language difficulties. A slightly higher refusal rate of 15 percent was encountered with respect to the controls. At the same time, a similar completion rate of 72 percent was experienced. Twelve percent of the control sample could not be reached because of changes in address or wrong telephone numbers. If we examine only the completed interviews and refusals, we encounter a 94 percent completion rate for cases and an 83 percent completion rate for controls.

Table 4.2 illustrates the interval between a caller initiating contact with the Can-Dial program and the subsequent interview. Most were contacted between one and three months after listening to the Can-Dial tape. During our early efforts, a number of individuals were interviewed about four months after making a call. However, we discovered that these people often had difficulty remembering the tape and the information they had received. For this reason, an effort was

Table 4.1 Interviews

	Callers		Controls	
	Number	Percent	Number	Percent
Complete interview	1,024	70.2	2,034	72.4
Refusals	64	4.4	419	14.9
Failure to contact	354	24.3	340	12.1
Partial interview	17	1.2	16	0.6
Total	1,459	100.1*	2,809	100.0

*Total differs from 100 percent due to rounding errors.

made to interview individuals within one or two months after their calling Can-Dial.

DEMOGRAPHIC CHARACTERISTICS

Significant differences between cases and controls were found in education, occupation, marital status, and age. A small difference was found in sex, the proportion of controls slightly favoring females compared to callers. No differences were found in urban, suburban,

Table 4.2 Interval between Contact and
Follow-up Interview

	Number	Percent
< 1 Month	6	0.5
1 Month	443	36.1
2 Months	359	29.2
3 Months	240	19.5
4 Months	138	11.2
Other	5	0.5
Total	1,191	100.0

Table 4.3 Demographic Characteristics: Callers and Controls

		Callers		Controls		χ^2 (P)
		Number	Percent	Number	Percent	
Education:	less than high school	160	15.8	285	27.8	
	high school	386	38.0	357	34.8	
	college	469	46.2	383	37.4	
Total		1,015	100.0	1,025	100.0	44.88 (P < 0.001)
Marital status:	married	783	77.1	732	71.5	
	single	197	19.4	149	13.8	
	widowed	35	3.5	151	14.7	
Total		1,015	100.0	1,024	100.0	83.30 (P < 0.001)
Age:	20–39	626	61.4	351	34.4	
	40–59	329	32.3	404	39.6	
	60 and over	64	6.3	265	26.0	
Total		1,019	100.0	1,020	100.0	207.88 (P < 0.001)
Sex:	females	739	72.5	805	79.8	
	males	281	27.5	204	20.2	
Total		1,020	100.0	1,009	100.0	14.99 (P < 0.001)
Occupation:	white-collar worker	376	40.0	314	36.7	
	blue-collar worker	389	41.3	308	36.0	
	unemployed worker	70	7.4	37	4.3	
	housewives and students	51	5.4	40	4.7	
	retiree	55	5.9	157	18.3	
Total		941	100.0	856	100.0	71.65 (P < 0.001)

Table 4.4 Health Awareness: Callers and Controls

		Callers		Controls		χ^2 (P)
		Number	Percent	Number	Percent	
Experience with cancer in significant others						
Friend or relative with cancer	Yes	774	76.3	666	65.8	
	No	240	23.7	346	34.2	
Total		1,014	100.0	1,012	100.0	27.27 (P < 0.001)
Relatives with cancer	0	416	40.9	524	51.5	
	1–4	602	59.1	494	48.5	
Total		1,018	100.0	1,018	100.0	23.05 (P < 0.001)
Total acquaintances with cancer	0	251	24.5	352	34.3	
	1–4	773	75.5	673	65.7	
Total		1,024	100.0	1,025	100.0	23.83 (P < 0.001)
Personal health and illness experience						
Physician visits in past year for illness	0	125	12.3	154	15.1	
	1–2	508	50.4	401	39.3	
	3 or more	376	37.3	466	45.6	
Total		1,009	100.0	1,021	100.0	25.16 (P < 0.001)
Smoker (ever)	Yes	736	72.5	618	60.4	
	No	279	27.5	405	39.6	
Total		1,015	100.0	1,023	100.0	33.46 (P < 0.001)
Types of health problems	Possibly cancer	140	38.7	65	16.6	
	Other	222	61.3	327	83.4	
Total		362	100.0	392	100.0	46.40 (P < 0.001)

or rural residence or socioeconomic status as derived from the census tract of residence.

Table 4.3 shows that cases had completed more education than controls: almost 28 percent of the controls compared to 16 percent of the callers terminated their schooling before finishing high school. Since education is often used as one indicator of social status, this may imply higher social class and greater sophistication about health matters that sometimes seems to coincide with higher levels of education. Regarding marital status, callers were also more likely than controls to be married and less likely to be widowed.

When head of household's occupation was examined, it was found that a significantly greater number of controls were retired. No interesting differences between other occupational groups were found. This result complements the findings that more controls than callers were widowed and that more controls than callers were over the age of 60. Our previous investigations showed greater use of the program by younger age groups, with older age groups demonstrating very low utilization. In view of the increase in risk with increasing age for most types of cancer, this lower use by older people is disturbing. These findings are also important since they emphasize the influence that age seems to exert in determining use of such programs and suggests that additional cancer control approaches need to be developed for the elderly.

HEALTH AWARENESS

Table 4.4 presents findings concerning the relationship between health awareness and Can-Dial use. Examination of respondents' experience with cancer revealed that more callers than controls reported having known someone with the disease, specifically having family members who had had cancer, and in general having known more cancer patients. Significant differences between cases and controls also were found for the number of friends who had experienced cancer.

In considering personal health and illness experience, it was discovered that controls exceeded callers in regular visits to their physician during a year's time. This finding probably reflects the tendency for controls to be older than callers and perhaps victims of more ailments requiring visits to a physician for treatment. No significant differences were found in number of nights spent in hospitals, although controls tended to exceed callers, or in the number of friends or relatives working in one of the health fields.

However, an interesting difference was found concerning smoking behavior, although in the opposite direction from that hypothesized. We had predicted that utilizers would display more health awareness than controls by being nonsmokers or ex-smokers. No

Table 4.5 Use of Media: Callers and Controls

Contact with Mass Media		Callers		Controls		χ^2 (P)
		Number	Percent	Number	Percent	
TV stations regularly watched	1	346	34.1	336	32.8	
	2-3	312	30.7	421	41.1	
	4	357	35.2	267	26.1	
Total		1,015	100.0	1,024	100.0	29.30 (P < 0.001)
Newspapers regularly read	0	138	13.5	81	7.9	
	1	417	40.8	385	37.6	
	2	467	45.7	558	54.5	
Total		1,022	100.0	1,024	100.0	24.19 (P < 0.001)

difference between ex-smokers was found. More cases than controls, however, reported that they were smoking or had done so in the past. Such an association is plausible when one recognizes the concern that has arisen regarding smoking during the past decade or so. Since our previous findings have shown topics concerning smoking to be among the most popular, it seems reasonable to assume that callers who smoked were concerned about their habit and therefore, even though they were engaged in an unhealthy activity, perhaps were aware of its health consequences, which prompted their contacting the system.

It was hypothesized that callers would be more likely to use the program than noncallers since the former would be more concerned about their health. However, no interesting differences between callers and controls were found in current health status or the presence of health problems. Only when health problems were grouped into those that might prompt one to be suspicious of cancer were differences found. As might be expected, callers exceeded controls in mentioning problems that prompted suspicion of cancer, whereas controls more often cited other types of health problems.

USE OF MEDIA

Table 4.5 presents findings regarding use of two forms of media. Callers were found to watch regularly a greater variety of television stations than controls. On the other hand, controls tended to be more regular newspaper readers than callers. No differences were found in frequency of watching television, frequency of reading newspapers, number of magazines regularly read, or frequency of reading magazine articles by physicians. A trend did exist for callers to listen to the radio more often and to more stations than did controls, although the difference was small.

KNOWLEDGE OF THE SEVEN DANGER SIGNALS

A major interest in evaluating the Can-Dial program was to ascertain the knowledge obtained from or changes in behavior resulting from contact with the system. The amount of knowledge was too varied to be investigated in a detailed manner in the interview time available; hence we compared the ability of cases and controls to state correctly the seven danger signals. Although this is an admittedly crude measure, it would suffice for providing some indication of the extent of simple, factual information retained that could influence preventive health behavior. Note in Table 4.6 that larger propor-

Table 4.6 Knowledge of Individual Danger Signals: Callers and Controls

		Callers		Controls		
	Response	Number	Percent	Number	Percent	χ^2 (P)
Sore that does not heal	Correct	470	46.0	379	37.0	
	Wrong	551	54.0	646	63.0	
Total		1,021	100.0	1,025	100.0	17.29 (P < 0.001)
Lump	Correct	714	69.7	682	66.5	
	Wrong	310	30.3	343	33.5	
Total		1,024	100.0	1,025	100.0	2.40 (NS)
Unusual bleeding or discharge	Correct	591	57.8	516	50.3	
	Wrong	432	42.2	509	49.7	
Total		1,023	100.0	1,025	100.0	11.38 (P < 0.001)
Change in bladder or bowel habits	Correct	290	28.3	235	22.9	
	Wrong	733	71.7	790	77.1	
Total		1,023	100.0	1,025	100.0	7.89 (P < 0.01)
Difficulty swallowing	Correct	86	8.4	72	7.0	
	Wrong	937	91.6	953	93.0	
Total		1,023	100.0	1,025	100.0	1.37 (NS)
Change in a wart or mole	Correct	310	30.3	234	22.8	
	Wrong	713	69.7	791	77.2	
Total		1,023	100.0	1,025	100.0	14.66 (P < 0.001)
Persistent cough	Correct	466	45.6	372	36.3	
	Wrong	557	54.4	652	63.7	
Total		1,023	100.0	1,024	100.0	18.01 (P < 0.001)

tions of both callers and noncallers recognized that a lump is characteristic of cancer. In view of the long-term publicity given the danger signals by the American Cancer Society, it seems remarkable that such a small percentage of respondents recognized such symptoms as difficulty in swallowing, change in a wart or mole, altered bowel habits, or a lesion that does not heal.

Slightly larger percentages of callers, ranging from 1 to 9 percent, were able to recognize each symptom, and 12 percent more callers than controls could recognize at least two danger signals. It could be argued that this constitutes evidence of successful retention of information obtained from the Can-Dial program. On the other hand, since we were unable to interview callers before they heard the Can-Dial information tapes, it could also be argued that they were more likely to be concerned about and aware of such matters than noncallers and consequently would possess more knowledge about cancer even prior to contact with the Can-Dial system.

PREVENTIVE HEALTH ORIENTATION

It was hypothesized that cases would be more likely than controls to display behavior reflecting a preventive health orientation. Therefore, we would expect them to demonstrate superior behavior over controls regarding the frequency of Pap tests, breast self-examination, physicians' visits for routine physical examinations, or yearly chest X-rays.

Table 4.7 indicates that, in addition to possessing more knowledge about cancer, callers exhibited behavior more oriented toward cancer prevention and control. Thus, they were more likely to have routine Pap tests, examine their breasts, and visit physicians for routine examinations, and a larger percentage had advised someone else to see a physician. These are the types of behavior we would like to see engendered by Can-Dial. It is possible that the contact callers had contributed to this behavior. It is also possible that other aspects of their experience, e.g., the publicity that accompanied the Rockefeller and Ford mastectomies, may have heightened their awareness. Moreover, we have no way of knowing whether or not the orientation exhibited by this behavior was present prior to or indeed may have prompted the call to Can-Dial. No differences were found in having heard of breast self-examination, having done breast self-examination, having heard of the Pap test, or the frequency of having chest X-rays.

Table 4.7 Preventive Health Care Orientation: Callers and Controls

		Callers		Controls		χ^2 (P)
		Number	Percent	Number	Percent	
Pap test	Once a year or more often	572	85.1	518	71.5	
	Less often than once a year	100	14.9	206	28.5	37.51 (P < 0.001)
Total		672	100.0	724	100.0	
Breast self-examination	Once a month or more often	364	55.3	361	47.6	
	Every few months	127	19.3	121	16.0	
	Occasionally or never	167	25.4	276	36.4	20.02 (P < 0.001)
Total		658	100.0	758	100.0	
Physician visits in past year for routine checkups	0	145	16.1	237	24.9	
	1–2	591	65.6	452	47.4	
	3–6	165	18.3	264	27.7	62.12 (P < 0.001)
Total		901	100.0	953	100.0	
Recent advice to some-one to see a physician	Yes	531	53.3	438	44.7	
	No	466	46.7	541	55.3	14.35 (P < 0.001)
Total		997	100.0	979	100.0	

CONCLUSION

In this chapter and the previous one, we have found that people who called the Can-Dial cancer information facility were better educated, younger, married individuals who were likely to have known family or friends who had cancer, were more likely to be smokers who had visited their physicians for routine checkups, and tended to watch more television stations, whereas noncallers tended to read more newspapers. Callers tended to discuss health topics with a more varied audience and were able to state correctly more of the seven warning signals than noncallers. These data provide qualified support for expectations that callers were more aware of health matters than noncallers, were more preventively oriented, differed in media consumption, and were more interested in health. They also demonstrate that those who contacted the program had more basic knowledge about cancer than noncallers, which may be viewed as evidence of the program's success.

Limitations of cancer information services such as Can-Dial are also suggested. The widowed, elderly, and less-educated have to be approached through different means, as do males in general. Increased efforts are required to make people more aware of the benefits of a preventive health orientation compared to a problem orientation. Obvious starting points are to employ existing educational facilities at places of work and organizations catering to older people, as well as hospitals and physicians' offices. It should be remembered that dial-access systems complement rather than supplant the educational activities of health professionals. The concern demonstrated by smokers suggests that continued and perhaps even increased efforts toward operation of smoking clinics and other smoking dissuasion efforts are warranted. However, dial-access systems alone probably do little by themselves to stop smoking in view of its addictive nature. Finally, information activities via the printed media, such as question-and-answer columns, short articles, and perhaps even regular syndicated columns, might appeal to that portion of the public more predisposed to print than oral and electronic media.

5

COMPARISON OF CALLERS WITH AND WITHOUT HEALTH PROBLEMS

In the previous two chapters we have examined the characteristics of callers and the patterns of their response, and compared the characteristics of callers with noncaller controls. In this chapter we are concerned with examining possible differences between callers with and those without health problems. Presence or absence of health problems was determined from responses to a question on current health status. We were interested in such possible differences since we hypothesized that Can-Dial users would be more likely to use the system if they were experiencing some type of illness.

MOTIVATION

When callers with and without problems were compared with respect to reasons for calling, no differences were found, as is demonstrated in Table 5.1. However, when these responses were grouped in the manner of Table 5.2, some interesting differences were observed. After responses concerning quitting smoking and those falling in the "other" category are eliminated, callers without problems show a tendency to fall in the "curious" category, whereas those with problems are more likely to have experienced illness themselves or in their family. This finding provides support for the notion that experience with cancer or current experience with a variety of health problems may have motivated some individuals to use the program.

Table 5.1 Reasons for Calling: Callers with and without
         Health Problems

	Callers with Problems		Callers without Problems	
	Number	Percent	Number	Percent
Desire to quit smoking	100	22.3	166	22.5
Curiosity	80	17.8	167	22.6
Cancer patient	11	2.5	7	1.0
Cancer in family	38	8.5	71	9.6
Other illness in family	7	1.6	18	2.4
Friend with cancer	12	2.7	15	2.0
Possible cancer symptoms	23	5.1	31	4.2
Desire for more knowledge	49	10.9	99	13.4
Current medical problem	70	15.6	49	6.6
Interest in a specific topic	39	8.7	82	11.1
Other	20	4.5	33	4.5
Total	449	100.2*	738	99.9*

*Total differs from 100 percent due to rounding errors.

Table 5.2 Motivation for Calling

	Callers with Problems		Callers without Problems	
	Number	Percent	Number	Percent
Curiosity	168	42.1	348	65.5
Illness in family	127	31.8	96	18.1
Personal illness	104	26.1	87	16.4
Total	399	100.0	531	100.0

Note: $\chi^2 = 50.90$, $P < 0.001$, 2 df

DEMOGRAPHIC CHARACTERISTICS

Significant differences between cases with health problems compared to those without were found in education, marital status, age,
sex, and socioeconomic status. Unlike the comparisons of cases with
noncaller controls mentioned in the previous chapter, no occupational
differences were found.

Table 5.3 shows that callers without problems had completed
more education than those with problems. Almost 23 percent of those
with problems had terminated their schooling before completing high
school compared to 9 percent of those without. This may indicate
that services such as Can-Dial serve as a resource for the less educated who experience medical problems. At the same time, better-
educated individuals may be more likely to employ services such as
Can-Dial when no illness is currently being experienced. This may
result from a greater preventive orientation among the better educated, with a consequent tendency for these individuals to call before
actually experiencing some kind of illness. The less educated, however, may have limited resources for obtaining information about
various types of health problems they encounter. Consequently, they
may have to turn to services such as telephone information programs
in order to obtain needed information. At the same time, it seems
the less educated are not as likely to use the program before an
actual illness is experienced.

With respect to marital status, a greater proportion of married
callers were not experiencing problems, whereas a larger percentage
of the formerly married were. This may be an age-related phenom-
enon since the formerly married are likely to be older than the currently married. At the same time, it may also jibe with previous
studies showing younger people to be more preventively oriented and
more open to accepting various types of innovations.

A tendency was observed for callers without problems to be
located in the age groups under 40. On the other hand, callers with
problems tended to be 50 years of age and over. Whether this is
largely the result of the effect of age upon health or whether it also
demonstrates a tendency for the elderly to make less use of telephone
information programs is difficult to determine at this time. However,
these findings support previous data showing Can-Dial callers to be
young, with those in the older age groups making less frequent use of
the program.

It was previously shown that females called approximately twice
as often as males. Upon examining the sex distribution of those with
and without problems, an increased tendency was found for males
without problems to call compared to males with problems. On the
other hand, females with problems exceeded those without, although

Table 5.3 Demographic Characteristics: Callers with and without Health Problems

		Callers with Problems		Callers without Problems		
		Number	Percent	Number	Percent	χ^2 (P)
Education:	0–11 years	106	22.9	70	9.3	
	12 years	180	38.9	294	39.0	
	More than 12 years	177	38.2	390	51.7	
Total		463	100.0	754	100.0	47.96 (P < 0.001)
Marital status:	Married	342	84.0	578	93.7	
	Formerly married	65	16.0	39	6.3	
Total		407	100.0	617	100.0	25.03 (P < 0.001)
Age:	20–39	110	23.8	373	49.2	
	40–59	215	46.5	288	38.0	
	60 and over	137	29.7	97	12.8	
Total		462	100.0	758	100.0	94.38 (P < 0.001)
Sex:	Male	104	22.5	231	30.6	
	Female	359	77.5	523	69.4	
Total		463	100.0	754	100.0	9.61 (P < 0.01)
Socioeconomic status:	Quartiles 1 and 2 (High)	235	50.4	451	59.3	
	Quartiles 3 and 4 (Low)	231	49.6	309	40.7	
Total		466	100.0	760	100.0	9.30 (P < 0.01)

Table 5.4 Socioeconomic Status: Callers with and without
Health Problems, Controlled for Residence

Residence	Quartile	Callers with Problems		Callers without Problems	
		Number	Percent	Number	Percent
Urban	1 (High)	66	32.5	96	36.4
	2	47	23.2	68	25.8
	3	57	28.1	67	25.4
	4 (Low)	33	16.3	33	12.5
Total		203 (46.8)	100.1*	264 (38.8)	100.1*
Suburban	1	49	28.5	96	31.1
	2	41	23.8	66	21.4
	3	36	20.9	80	25.9
	4	46	26.7	67	21.7
Total		172 (39.6)	99.9*	309 (45.4)	100.1*
Rural	1	16	27.1	24	22.4
	2	17	28.8	33	30.8
	3	13	22.0	28	26.2
	4	13	22.0	22	20.6
Total		59 (13.6)	99.9*	107 (15.7)	100.0
		434 (100.0)		680 (99.9)*	

*Total differs from 100 percent due to rounding errors.
Note: Marginal $\chi^2 = 6.88$, $P < 0.05$, 2 df

once again differences were small. Even though definitive conclusions
cannot be made on the basis of these data, it is possible to speculate
that males currently experiencing health problems might be less
likely than females to make use of public information facilities. Since
a large portion of male callers were interested in smoking-related
topics, these data may reflect male concern about the health effects
of smoking. Hence, rather than using telephone information programs
as a general health resource, males may be interested only in specific topics. Alternative methods need to be devised for reaching
males in order to promote other forms of improved health and cancer
control behavior.

Previous comparisons of cases and noncaller controls did not
show any socioeconomic differences. However, when socioeconomic

Table 5.5 Health Awareness: Callers with and without Health Problems

		Callers with Problems		Callers without Problems		
		Number	Percent	Number	Percent	χ^2 (P)
Experience with cancer in significant others						
Friend with cancer	Yes	376	81.2	547	72.6	
	No	87	18.8	206	27.4	
Total		463	100.0	753	100.0	11.51 (P < 0.001)
Relatives with cancer	0	175	37.6	315	41.4	
	1	158	33.9	276	36.3	
	More than 1	133	28.5	169	22.2	
Total		466	100.0	760	99.9*	4.36 (NS)
Total acquaintances with cancer	0	91	19.5	213	28.0	
	1 or more	375	80.5	547	72.0	
Total		466	100.0	760	100.0	11.19 (P < 0.001)
Personal health and illness experience						
Physician visits in past year for illness	0–3	230	50.2	649	86.2	
	4 or more	228	49.8	104	13.8	
Total		458	100.0	753	100.0	185.17 (P < 0.001)
Time in hospitals	0	16	3.5	91	12.2	
	Less than 1 month	247	54.4	210	28.2	
	1 month or more	191	42.1	445	59.6	
Total		454	100.0	746	100.0	91.36 (P < 0.001)

*Total differs from 100 percent due to rounding errors.

status for callers with and without problems was investigated, small but interesting differences were found. Table 5.3 shows a tendency for callers without problems to exceed those with problems in the two highest socioeconomic quartiles. By the same token, callers with problems exceeded those without them in the two lowest quartiles. These findings parallel those concerning education in that low SES individuals were more likely to utilize the Can-Dial program when a health problem was currently being experienced. On the other hand, those of high socioeconomic status were more likely to make use of the problem for informational purposes before a health problem was experienced, if one assumes they were responding honestly with respect to experiencing health problems.

Since residence was previously found related to response, utilization for those with problems compared to those without by socioeconomic quartile was examined when residence was controlled. No SES differences were found. Small differences were found in residence when the marginal totals were examined. Among urban dwellers, a larger percentage reported experiencing problems, whereas among suburbanites a larger proportion did not mention experiencing any. No differences were found in rural dwellers (see Table 5.4).

HEALTH AWARENESS

Differences among callers with and without problems with respect to health awareness were also examined. Table 5.5 shows small but suggestive differences in response to a question about acquaintance with cancer patients. More callers with problems answered positively as compared to those without problems. Suggestive findings were also encountered for having experienced cancer in one's family, callers with problems exceeding those without.

Finally, when the total number of friends or relatives who had cancer was examined, callers with problems were found to exceed those without them. These findings suggest that callers who experienced health problems were also more likely to have known someone who had cancer.

Personal health and illness experience can also be an important motivating factor. Fifty percent of cases with problems were found to have visited physicians four or more times in the preceding year compared to 14 percent of those without problems. At the same time, 86 percent of those without problems visited physicians three or fewer times during the preceding year as opposed to 50 percent of those with problems. However, investigation of the number of nights spent in hospitals showed more callers without problems to have spent more than one month in a hospital. Sixty percent of those without

Table 5.6 Preventive Health Care Orientation: Callers with and without Health Problems

	Callers with Problems		Callers without Problems		χ^2 (P)
	Number	Percent	Number	Percent	
Physician visits in past year					
for routine checkups					
0–2	275	69.8	603	89.9	
3 or more	119	30.2	68	10.1	69.07 (P < 0.001)
Total	394	100.0	671	100.0	
Recent advice to someone					
to see a physician					
Yes	271	60.2	364	49.3	
No	179	39.8	375	50.7	13.52 (P < 0.001)
Total	450	100.0	739	100.0	

problems spent more than one month in a hospital compared to 42 percent of those with problems. At the same time, 54 percent of those
cases with problems stated they had spent less than a month in hospitals as opposed to 28 percent of those without problems.

PREVENTIVE HEALTH ORIENTATION

Earlier case control comparisons showed callers to have had
a Pap test more often, to have conducted breast self-examination
more frequently, and to have had more checkups than noncallers. No
differences were found among callers with problems as compared to
those without in frequency of having Pap tests or doing breast self-
examination. However, when visits to physicians for routine checkups
were examined (Table 5.6) approximately 90 percent of callers without
problems were found to have seen their physician fewer than two
times in the past year. On the other hand, 30 percent of those with
problems visited their physicians three or more times as compared
to 10 percent of the callers without problems. This information may
be biased because of age or because interviewers did not make clear
the purpose of this question. People with a chronic problem such as
hypertension are likely to visit their physicians routinely for blood
pressure monitoring, which could be viewed as a routine checkup.
Older individuals would also be more likely to fall into this category.
In response to the question "Have you told anyone to see a doctor recently?" 60 percent of the callers with problems answered in
the affirmative as opposed to 49 percent of those without. This cor-
responds with previous findings concerning differences between callers and noncaller controls. When questioned as to why they advised
someone to see a physician, 61 percent of the callers with problems
cited poor health compared to 51 percent of those without problems.
At the same time, 37 percent of cases without problems as opposed
to 29 percent of those with them cited immediate illness as a reason.
These last findings may indicate a tendency for callers with problems
to be more vocal about health as opposed to those without.
We did not find any differences between callers with and without
problems with respect to media use or knowledge of the seven danger
signals. Such findings are interesting since they imply that communication patterns are not affected by the presence or absence of health
problems. They also show that knowledge of cancer as measured by
the seven danger signals is not influenced by health problems.

CONCLUSION

In this chapter we have attempted to distinguish between callers with some kind of health problem and those without so as to ascertain any differences in characteristics that might affect use of the program. Many of the findings cited parallel those reported in the previous chapter with respect to differences between callers and noncaller controls. We found differences in demographic characteristics such as education, marital status, age, and socioeconomic status. We also found some differences with respect to indicators of health awareness and personal health and illness experience. Small suggestive differences were found in preventive health orientation. The fact that no differences in media use were discovered indicates that callers were probably similar in their communication patterns. Absence of differences in knowledge as measured by the seven danger signals may imply that receiving information from the program affected knowledge more than presence or absence of illness. The next chapter will be concerned with comparing cases and controls with suspected cancer symptoms.

6

COMPARISON OF CALLERS
AND CONTROLS WITH
POSSIBLE CANCER PROBLEMS

Earlier attempts to investigate health problems experienced by cases and controls revealed no differences in frequency, total number, or types of health problems experienced. However, when health problems were grouped into those that might raise the suspicion of cancer, some interesting differences between cases and controls were observed. This chapter is concerned with describing results of comparisons of cases and controls with problems suggestive of cancer.

DEMOGRAPHIC CHARACTERISTICS

Significant differences were observed in education, marital status, age, and occupation (Table 6.1). No differences were found in sex or socioeconomic status. A much larger proportion of noncaller controls possessed less than a high school education when compared to cases. However, 46.2 percent of the cases as compared to 29 percent of the controls had at least a high school education. A slightly larger percentage of callers than controls had attended college, although the difference was only about 3 percent. These findings show that Can-Dial was used more by better-educated individuals who experienced health problems that might arouse the suspicion of cancer. Thus, among those who were experiencing possible cancer-related health problems, those who are somewhat better educated may be more likely to utilize telephone cancer information services. This finding coincides with our previous findings regarding Can-Dial use and education.

When marital status was examined, 82 percent of the callers and 66 percent of the controls were found to be married. At the same

Table 6.1 Demographic Characteristics: Callers and Controls with Possible Cancer Symptoms

		Callers		Controls		χ^2 (P)
		Number	Percent	Number	Percent	
Education	Less than high school	39	21.2	86	41.6	
	High school	85	46.2	61	29.4	
	College	60	32.6	60	29.0	
Total		184	100.0	207	100.0	20.34 (P < 0.001)
Marital status	Married	148	81.8	136	66.3	
	Widowed	8	4.4	45	22.0	
	Single	25	13.8	24	11.7	
Total		181	100.0	205	100.0	24.96 (P < 0.001)
Age	20-39	92	49.7	37	17.6	
	40-59	75	40.5	97	46.2	
	60 and over	18	9.7	76	36.2	
Total		185	99.9*	210	100.0	60.71 (P < 0.001)
Occupation	Retiree	16	8.9	37	20.3	
	Other	164	91.1	145	79.7	
Total		180	100.0	182	100.0	9.48 (P < 0.01)

*Total differs from 100 percent due to rounding errors.

54

time, 22 percent of the controls compared to 4 percent of the cases were widowed. It is interesting that a much larger proportion of callers with possible cancer symptoms than controls were married. The increased proportion of widowed individuals among controls may be due in part to the slightly higher age of controls. Even so, this probably could not account for the large caller-control differences observed here. The greater likelihood for married individuals who are experiencing cancer symptoms to employ the Can-Dial program suggests that married people may be more aware and more concerned about health matters than individuals who have lost their spouse.* A need for increased activities oriented toward the widowed is suggested. These not only need to be supportive in many different senses of the term but also should include active attempts to stimulate individuals to be more aware and more concerned about their health. Information programs such as Can-Dial need to develop efforts oriented specifically toward these groups.

Examination of the age characteristics of callers and controls with possible cancer symptoms revealed differences similar to those previously found. Callers tended to be younger than controls. In fact, just under 75 percent of the callers were under 50 compared to approximately 36 percent of the controls. Among those experiencing health problems that might be cancer-related, younger people were more likely to use the program than those who were older. Once again, this supports our previous contentions that special efforts need to be directed toward the elderly.

Investigation of occupation yielded few differences between callers and controls. The only interesting differences were found among those who were retired. As would be expected in light of the age difference we have just reported, controls exceeded callers among the retired. This may be important since we suspect that a basic prerequisite for contacting the Can-Dial program was time available in which to make the telephone call. Retired individuals are more likely to have sufficient time than are those who are actively working. Therefore, one would not expect lack of time to exert a significant influence in this case. More likely, a lack of interest in the program probably accounted for these differences among the retired.

---

*Studies of bereavement have suggested that widows and widowers are more likely to experience increased morbidity and mortality from a variety of causes. Perhaps a decreased interest in health is involved, which could parallel our experience with Can-Dial.

Table 6.2 Health Awareness: Callers and Controls with Possible Cancer Symptoms

Experience with Cancer in Significant Others		Callers		Controls		χ^2 (P)
		Number	Percent	Number	Percent	
Friend or relative with cancer	Yes	159	86.4	154	75.1	
	No	25	13.6	51	24.9	7.86 (P < 0.01)
Total		184	100.0	205	100.0	
Friends with cancer	0	119	64.3	155	74.2	
	1–4	66	35.7	54	25.8	4.49 (P < 0.05)
Total		185	100.0	209	100.0	
Relatives with cancer	0	56	30.3	87	41.4	
	1	64	34.6	73	34.8	
	2 or more	65	35.1	50	23.8	7.72 (P < 0.05)
Total		185	100.0	210	100.0	
Total acquaintances with cancer	0	25	13.5	53	25.2	
	1	71	38.4	84	40.0	
	2 or more	89	48.1	73	34.8	11.18 (P < 0.01)
Total		185	100.0	210	100.0	
Friends working in health fields	0	144	77.8	182	86.7	
	1 or more	41	22.2	28	13.3	5.32 (P < 0.05)
Total		185	100.0	210	100.0	

These findings may be associated with the effects of age. At
the same time, they may provide clues to reasons why the elderly
seemed less interested and made less use of the Can-Dial program
than younger individuals.

Although age has been found related to use of Can-Dial, other
factors such as amount of education, current marital status, and
occupation also influence decisions to seek further information about
health. Additional research is needed to determine how these and
other characteristics affect decisions to utilize health information
programs.

HEALTH AWARENESS

As previously mentioned, it was hypothesized that individuals
possessing greater health awareness would be more likely to utilize
the Can-Dial program than those less concerned about health. Table
6.2 presents findings concerning the relationship between health
awareness and Can-Dial use for those with health problems that might
lead one to suspect cancer. It was found that callers with cancer
symptoms were more likely to have known several cancer patients
than controls with these symptoms. Likewise, when questioned as to
the number of friends who had experienced cancer, a larger portion
of controls with cancer symptoms responded in the negative. Callers
were more likely than controls to mention having known one or more
friends who had had the disease. Similarly, when we examined the
number of family members who had had cancer, more controls than
callers mentioned that no one in their family had ever experienced
cancer, whereas more callers than controls cited two or more of
their family as having had cancer. When the total number of cancer
acquaintances was examined, controls more often mentioned having
known no one with cancer than did callers. By the same token, more
callers than controls mentioned having known two or more friends,
relatives, or acquaintances who had had the disease.

Our previous investigations showed no relationship between
the number of friends or relatives working in health fields and Can-
Dial use. We had originally hypothesized that contact with such people
would help make one more aware of health matters and consequently
motivate individuals to use the Can-Dial program. However, our
previous analyses revealed no differences between cases and controls
in this respect. Table 6.1 demonstrates a tendency for cases with
cancer symptoms to cite more friends working in the health areas
than controls. It is possible that individuals who are experiencing
possible cancer-related health problems may be more aware of the
potential seriousness of their problems as a result of contact with

Table 6.3 Personal Health and Illness Experience: Callers and Controls with Possible Cancer Symptoms

	Callers		Controls		χ^2 (P)
	Number	Percent	Number	Percent	
Physician visits in past year for illness					
0	8	4.7	7	3.3	
1-3	56	33.1	66	31.6	
4 or more	105	62.1	136	65.1	
Total	169	99.9*	209	100.0	0.65 (NS)
Smoker (ever)					
Yes	136	73.5	134	64.1	
No	49	26.5	75	35.9	
Total	185	100.0	209	100.0	4.02 (P < 0.05)
Children living at home					
0	53	29.4	108	52.7	
1-2	77	42.8	65	31.7	
3 or more	50	27.8	32	15.6	
Total	180	100.0	205	100.0	22.23 (P < 0.001)

*Total differs from 100 percent due to rounding errors.

health workers. Consequently, this would have served as a motivating factor to use the system. Individuals who are experiencing health problems but at the same time do not have contact with health-allied workers either may be unaware of the possible seriousness of their problems or may not know about the availability of health information programs and the types of information available.

These results provide additional support for previous findings regarding the relationship between health awareness and Can-Dial use. Of those individuals currently experiencing health problems that might be cancer-related, those who gave evidence of possessing increased health awareness were more likely to utilize the Can-Dial program.

PERSONAL HEALTH AND ILLNESS EXPERIENCE

Earlier chapters provided evidence of the influence of personal health and illness experiences upon use of the Can-Dial program. For instance, comparisons of cases and controls showed a tendency for the former to have made one or two visits to their physician during the preceding year because of illness, whereas controls more often than cases cited making three or more such visits. When we investigated this same variable for callers and controls with possible cancer symptoms, we found no differences, as is illustrated by Table 6.3. This suggests that among the subpopulation of callers and controls with cancer symptoms, contact with physicians because of illness did not discriminate between cases and controls or perhaps was irrelevant under the circumstances.

Examination of smoking behavior shows that a greater proportion of cases than controls with cancer symptoms responded that they had at some time smoked, and that more controls said they had never smoked when compared to cases. When asked if they had stopped smoking, a larger percentage of controls than cases answered in the affirmative. Although the differences were small, when they are viewed in light of the popularity of smoking-related topics and the previous findings concerning differences between callers and noncallers, it becomes evident that smoking was probably more of a motivating factor to use Can-Dial than experience with cancer-related problems.

During the interviews, we asked about the number of children currently living at home. We had hypothesized that individuals with children at home would be more likely to make use of the Can-Dial program since they would be more likely to be aware of and concerned about health problems. Comparisons of callers and noncallers revealed virtually no differences, as did comparisons of callers with

Table 6.4 Use of Media: Callers and Controls with Possible Cancer Symptoms

		Callers		Controls		
		Number	Percent	Number	Percent	χ^2 (P)
TV stations regularly watched	0–2	95	51.4	100	47.6	
	3–4	51	27.6	93	44.3	
	More than 4	39	21.1	17	8.1	
Total		185	100.1*	210	100.0	19.52 (P < 0.001)
Newspapers regularly read	0–1	114	62.3	100	47.6	
	2 or more	69	37.7	110	52.4	
Total		183	100.0	210	100.0	8.49 (P < 0.01)
Magazines regularly read	0–1	119	64.7	154	72.6	
	2	48	26.1	30	14.2	
	3 or more	17	9.2	28	13.2	
Total		184	100.0	212	100.0	9.39 (P < 0.01)

*Total differs from 100 percent due to rounding errors.

and without symptoms. However, when those with cancer symptoms were examined, we do see some interesting differences. A much greater proportion of controls stated that they had no children living at home, whereas significantly larger numbers of callers answered in the affirmative. Undoubtedly, age is a factor, since in our society the elderly are less likely to have children living at home than are individuals 50 and under. This observation tends to support our hypothesis that families with children are more likely to be aware of health problems and consequently more likely to utilize programs such as Can-Dial.

MEDIA USE

Previous analyses showed significant differences between callers and noncallers for certain items pertaining to use of media. Specifically, callers watched a greater variety of television stations than controls, and, at the same time, controls read more newspapers than callers. Examination of cases and controls with possible cancer problems revealed similar findings, as shown in Table 6.4. Callers reported that they regularly watched more television stations than did controls. Likewise, once again controls reported reading more newspapers than callers. These findings support earlier results and suggest that differences in media use continue even when cancer-related health problems are experienced. However, in addition, significant differences were found for the number of magazines read. A greater percentage of callers with cancer symptoms reported reading two magazines compared to controls with such symptoms. These findings may indicate greater reliance by controls upon local information sources such as local newspapers, whereas callers were more attuned to more cosmopolitan sources of printed information, such as magazines. It would be fruitful for future investigators to investigate differences in communication patterns and their relationship to use of health-related innovations in greater detail.

PREVENTIVE HEALTH ORIENTATION

We had hypothesized that individuals who were more preventively oriented would make greater use of the Can-Dial program than those who were not. Some evidence in support of this contention was provided in Chapter 4. For instance, callers more frequently had Pap tests, did breast self-examinations, and visited physicians for routine checkups, and they were more likely to have advised someone to see a physician. Similar results were obtained upon examining callers

Table 6.5 Preventive Health Care Orientation: Callers and Controls with Possible Cancer Symptoms

		Callers		Controls		
		Number	Percent	Number	Percent	χ^2 (P)
Pap tests	Never	1	0.8	16	10.5	
	Less often than once a year	11	8.5	27	17.8	
	Once a year or more often	117	90.7	109	71.7	
Total		129	100.0	152	100.0	18.50 (P < 0.001)
Breast self-examination	Never	15	11.6	43	26.2	
	Less often than once a month	45	34.9	38	23.2	
	At least once a month or after period	69	53.5	83	50.6	
Total		129	100.0	164	100.0	11.38 (P < 0.01)
Chest X-rays	When required by employer or doctor	11	6.5	36	18.8	
	Less often than every three years	58	34.3	42	21.9	
	Every three years or more often	100	59.2	114	59.4	
Total		169	100.0	192	100.1*	15.37 (P < 0.001)
Physician visits in past year for routine checkups	None	24	14.8	29	15.1	
	Three times or less	92	56.8	74	38.5	
	More than three times	46	28.4	89	46.4	
Total		162	100.0	192	100.0	13.68 (P < 0.01)
Recent advice to someone to see a physician	Yes	108	59.3	88	43.6	
	No	74	40.7	114	56.4	
Total		182	100.0	202	100.0	9.54 (P < 0.01)

*Total differs from 100 percent due to rounding errors.

62

and controls with possible cancer problems. Table 6.5 shows that a greater percentage of callers with cancer problems reported having had Pap tests at least once a year compared to controls. Likewise, more controls than callers reported never having had a Pap test or having had them less often than once a year.

A greater percentage of callers reported practicing breast self-examination frequently than did controls. Twenty-six percent of the controls compared with about 12 percent of the callers reported that they never engaged in breast self-examination.

Table 6.5 demonstrates the frequency of obtaining chest X-rays. We found no differences between cases and controls who had had chest X-rays when required by their employer or doctor. However, 34 percent of the cases reported having chest X-rays less often than every three years as opposed to about 22 percent of the controls. Controls exceeded cases among those who reported receiving chest X-rays more often than every three years. Although not conclusive, this is the reverse of what we would expect if frequent chest X-rays are evidence of a greater preventive orientation.

When frequency of visits to physicians for routine checkups was investigated, 57 percent of the callers reported three or fewer during the preceding year as compared to 38 percent of the controls. Forty-six percent of the controls as compared to 28 percent of the callers mentioned that they visited their physician more than three times during that period. In all probability, these responses indicate the presence of some kind of chronic problem that required frequent follow-up visits rather than a preventive orientation. This explanation is even more viable when one recognizes that this group was comprised entirely of individuals who mentioned having health problems that might be cancer-related.

That more callers responded in the affirmative to questions concerning having recently advised someone to see a physician reinforces earlier findings. Callers seem to be more interested in health matters, are more likely to advise someone to see a doctor, and at the same time seem to be more likely to talk about health-related topics than controls.

CONCLUSION

In this chapter, we have examined differences between cases and controls who experienced possible cancer-related health problems. For the most part, our findings are similar to those reported in Chapter 4. In some instances, increased differences between the two categories were found. This implies that the same factors associated with prompting individuals to call are present—usually to a somewhat stronger degree—when possible cancer-related health problems are being experienced. Although higher education, relative youth, greater awareness of health matters, use of media, and preventive orientation are important for distinguishing between users and nonusers, these characteristics seem even more pronounced among those who are experiencing health problems that might indicate cancer.

7

IMPACT OF THE PROGRAM

A major objective of this evaluation was to determine the immediate influence exerted by information received from the program upon callers' behavior. During the telephone interviews, callers were asked several questions aimed at determining action taken or changes in behavior that the listener attributed to contact with the Can-Dial program.

INFLUENCES UPON BEHAVIOR

Table 7.1 provides a breakdown of responses to the question "What did you do as a result of hearing the tape?" Approximately 40 percent reported taking no action, and 25 percent cited smoking-related changes including cutting down, quitting, changing brands, or attending a smoking clinic. Another 11 percent stated that they visited or made an appointment with a physician or a clinic. A variety of other responses were also received covering a rather wide range of categories.

If these responses are grouped in the manner of Table 7.2, we find them somewhat easier to interpret. Approximately 40 percent of the respondents adopted some type of positive health behavior as a result of contact with the Can-Dial system. This included smoking-related activities, visiting or making appointments with physicians, beginning breast self-examination, having Pap tests, or reducing exposure to the sun. Approximately 10 percent took positive but not necessarily health-related action. This included discussing information received from the program, using this information for various school projects, and so forth. Another group of reported behaviors

Table 7.1 Action Taken: All Callers, 1974–1976

	Response	
	Number	Percent
Reduction in smoking	149	14.6
Success in quitting smoking	49	4.8
Attempt to quit smoking/change of brands	52	5.1
Attendance at a smoking clinic	7	0.7
Doctor visit	91	8.9
Made appointment with physician	29	2.8
Breast self-examination	15	1.5
Pap test	5	0.5
Reduced exposure to sun	5	0.5
Discussion about cancer with family	51	5.0
Feeling of being informed	76	7.4
Reflection upon the information	19	1.9
Feeling of reassurance	15	1.5
Use of information for class project, research, etc.	12	1.2
Nothing	408	39.9
Other	40	3.9
Total	1,023	100.2*

*Total differs from 100 percent due to rounding errors.
Source: G. S. Wilkinson, E. A. Mirand, and S. Graham, Cancer Information by Telephone: A Two-Year Evaluation, Health Education Monographs, vol. 5, no. 3, pp. 251-65, 1977. Reprinted with permission of the Society for Public Health Education, Inc.

could be defined as positive in a passive sense in that no direct
activity was forthcoming. This includes reports that contact with
the program helped relieve anxiety, stimulated thinking about the
information received, or increased knowledge. Consequently,
whereas 40 percent of the callers did nothing in direct response to
contact with the program, another 40 percent adopted improved cancer control behavior. An additional 20 percent were positively affected. It should be kept in mind that these were relatively short-term
changes taking place less than six months and usually within two or
three months after contact with the system.

We were also interested in examining the influence upon behavior for individuals with compared to those without health-related
problems. Table 7.3 shows the distribution of responses when callers
were categorized in this manner. No large differences between these
two groups were found. A slightly larger percentage of callers with
problems reported cutting down on smoking or visiting their physician, while a somewhat larger percentage of those without problems
reported taking no action. If we group responses in the manner of
Table 7.4, we find that a larger proportion of callers with problems
than those without took positive health-related action, and that a
larger proportion of callers without problems than those with them
reported doing nothing. The differences, however, are so small that
no definite conclusions can be reached on the basis of these data
alone.

The diffusion of information obtained from the Can-Dial program
would be interesting to investigate especially with respect to changes

Table 7.2 Impact upon Behavior: All Callers, 1974-1976

	Response	
	Number	Percent
Positive, health-related impact	407	39.8
Postive impact, not health-related	98	9.6
Positive but passive impact	110	10.8
Negative or no impact	408	39.8
Total	1,023	100.0

Source: G. S. Wilkinson, E. A. Mirand, and S. Graham,
Cancer Information by Telephone: A Two-Year Evaluation, Health
Education Monographs, vol. 5, no. 3, pp. 251-65, 1977. Reprinted
with permission of the Society for Public Health Education, Inc.

Table 7.3 Action Taken: Callers with and without Health Problems

	Callers with Problems		Callers without Problems	
	Number	Percent	Number	Percent
Reduction in smoking	76	16.9	107	14.5
Success in quitting smoking	24	5.3	37	5.0
Attendance at a smoking clinic	1	0.2	2	0.3
Visit doctor	47	10.4	51	6.9
Made appointment with physician	11	2.4	25	3.4
Breast self-examination	5	1.1	13	1.8
Pap test	2	0.4	3	0.4
Discussion about cancer with family	20	4.4	35	4.8
Feeling of being informed	31	6.9	56	7.6
Feeling of reassurance	13	2.9	9	1.2
Nothing	174	38.6	316	42.9
Other	47	10.4	83	11.3
Total	451	99.9*	737	100.0

*Total differs from 100 percent due to rounding errors.

Table 7.4 Impact upon Behavior: Callers with and without Health Problems

	Callers with Problems		Callers without Problems	
	Number	Percent	Number	Percent
Positive, health-related impact	166	41.1	238	36.4
Positive impact, not health-related, or passive	64	15.8	100	15.3
Negative or no impact	174	43.1	316	48.3
Total	404	100.0	654	100.0

Note: $\chi^2 = 2.98$, NS

Table 7.5 Discussion of the Information
with Another Person

	Number	Percent
Yes	621	60.7
No	396	38.7
No answer/other	6	0.6
Total	1,023	100.0

in behavior on the part of respondents of the second order. Table 7.5 provides responses to questions as to whether callers talked to anyone about the information they received from the program. Sixty-one percent answered in the affirmative as opposed to 39 percent in the negative. This information in and of itself is interesting since it shows that a majority discussed the materials they were exposed to with others. It is through informal communication networks that considerable diffusion of information takes place. However, by itself, all this information tells us is that a majority of individuals interviewed who contacted the program passed some of this information on to others. Respondents were also asked if individuals with whom they discussed the information took any direct action in the form of making appointments or visiting their physicians or clinics. Between 11 and 12 percent answered affirmatively (Table 7.6). If these responses can be relied upon, they indicate an additional impact of the program—not upon individuals who contacted Can-Dial, but rather upon people with whom callers discussed the information. As such, it comprises an additional influence exerted by the system.

Table 7.6 Visits to a Physician or Clinic

	Number	Percent
Yes	46	11.6
No	345	87.1
Don't know	5	1.3
Total	396	100.0

Table 7.7 Knowledge of the Seven Danger Signals:
Callers and Controls

Total Correct Answers	Callers		Controls	
	Number	Percent	Number	Percent
0-1	224	21.9	321	31.3
2-3	428	41.8	416	40.6
More than 3	372	36.3	288	28.1
Total	1,024	100.0	1,025	100.0

Note: χ^2 = 28.16, P < 0.001

KNOWLEDGE

Knowledge is another possible indicator of program impact.
Cases would be expected to demonstrate more knowledge than controls about cancer, presumably as a result of contact with the program. Table 7.7 shows differences between the two regarding knowledge of the seven danger signals. As was reported in Chapter 4, cases
exceeded controls in the number of correct answers for all of the
seven danger signals. Although at times the differences between the
two groups were small, the same trend persists throughout.* When
the correct answers were grouped in the manner of Table 7.7, the
number of controls giving fewer than two of the danger signals correctly was found to exceed the number of callers who did so; callers
and controls were similar in citing two or three correctly; and more
callers than controls gave more than three correctly. These findings
may indicate greater knowledge on the part of callers as a result of
information obtained from the Can-Dial program. However, this conclusion must be qualified since we did not collect information pertaining to knowledge at the time of the call. If it had been possible to
collect such information, it would then be feasible to compare responses before and after listening to the information provided. Consequently, the differences between callers and controls demonstrated
in this table may also indicate that callers knew more about cancer
even before they called.

----

*Differences between callers and controls regarding knowledge
of the seven danger signals are reported in detail in Chapter 4. See
Table 4.6.

Table 7.8 Knowledge of the Seven Danger Signals: Callers with and without Health Problems

	Response	Callers with Problems		Callers without Problems		χ^2 (P)
		Number	Percent	Number	Percent	
Sore that does not heal	Wrong	254	54.5	406	53.6	
	Correct	212	45.5	351	46.4	0.09 (NS)
Lump	Wrong	128	27.5	246	32.4	
	Correct	338	72.5	514	67.6	3.27 (NS)
Unusual bleeding or discharge	Wrong	181	38.8	329	43.3	
	Correct	285	61.2	430	56.7	2.41 (NS)
Change in bowel or bladder habits	Wrong	316	67.8	559	73.6	
	Correct	150	32.2	200	26.4	4.82 (P < 0.05)
Difficulty swallowing	Wrong	411	88.2	705	92.8	
	Correct	55	11.8	54	7.2	7.83 (P < 0.01)
Change in a wart or mole	Wrong	324	69.5	523	68.8	
	Correct	142	30.5	236	31.2	0.05 (NS)
Persistent cough	Wrong	247	53.0	401	52.8	
	Correct	219	47.0	358	47.2	0.03 (NS)

Table 7.9 Knowledge of the Seven Danger Signals: Callers and Controls with Possible Cancer Symptoms

	Response	Callers with Cancer Symptoms		Controls with Cancer Symptoms		χ^2 (P)
		Number	Percent	Number	Percent	
Sore that does not heal	Wrong	91	49.2	132	63.2	
	Correct	94	50.8	77	36.8	7.80 (P < 0.01)
Lump	Wrong	44	23.8	73	34.9	
	Correct	141	76.2	136	65.1	5.84 (P < 0.05)
Unusual bleeding or discharge	Wrong	72	38.9	96	45.7	
	Correct	113	61.1	114	54.3	1.86 (NS)
Change in bowel or bladder habits	Wrong	117	63.2	155	73.8	
	Correct	68	36.8	55	26.2	5.12 (P < 0.05)
Difficulty swallowing	Wrong	163	88.1	192	91.4	
	Correct	22	11.9	18	8.6	1.19 (NS)
Change in a wart or mole	Wrong	126	68.1	159	75.7	
	Correct	59	31.9	51	24.3	2.83 (NS)
Persistent cough	Wrong	100	54.1	133	63.3	
	Correct	85	45.9	77	36.7	3.50 (NS)

It was hypothesized that callers with problems would be able to state correctly more of the seven danger signals than those without problems. Callers with problems would be more aware and more concerned about their health and therefore more likely to retain information gained from the program if they had not already obtained it before. However, as Table 7.8 shows, few differences were found between callers with and without problems with respect to each of the seven danger signals. In only two, those concerning changes in bowel habits and difficulty swallowing, did callers with problems exceed in number those without problems to a significant degree. Although the differences were statistically significant regarding change in bowel habits, only a 6 percent difference was found, and in the case of difficulty in swallowing, only a 4 percent difference. Consequently, we must conclude that the presence or absence of health problems does not influence knowledge to any significant extent as measured by the seven warning signals. However, when callers with cancer symptoms were compared to controls with cancer symptoms (table 7.9), several significant differences were discovered. Callers exceeded controls in number with respect to knowledge of sores that do not heal, the presence of lumps, and changes in bowel or bladder habits. For other danger signals, callers always exceeded controls although the differences were not statistically significant. When the information is grouped in the manner of Table 7.10, the tendency for callers with symptoms to be more numerous than controls with symptoms in the number of correct warning signals they cited becomes more evident. Twenty-two percent of the controls as opposed to 7 percent of the callers were unable to mention correctly any of the seven danger signals. Equal numbers of callers and controls correctly

Table 7.10 Knowledge of the Seven Danger Signals: Callers and Controls with Possible Cancer Symptoms

Total Correct Answers	Callers		Controls	
	Number	Percent	Number	Percent
0	14	7.6	46	21.9
1-2	48	26.0	56	26.7
3 or more	123	66.5	108	51.4
Total	185	100.1*	210	100.0

*Total differs from 100 percent due to rounding errors.
Note: χ^2 = 17.14, P < 0.001, 2 df

Table 7.11 Topic Selected and Knowledge of the Seven Danger Signals

	Selected	Correct		Incorrect		χ^2 (P)
		Number	Percent	Number	Percent	
Sore that does not heal	Yes	8	1.8	13	2.4	
	No	434	98.2	523	97.6	
Total		442	100.0	536	100.0	0.44 (NS)
Lump	Yes	108	16.3	32	10.1	
	No	555	83.7	286	89.9	
Total		663	100.0	318	100.0	6.81 (< 0.01)
Unusual bleeding or discharge	Yes	49	8.8	17	4.1	
	No	511	91.3	403	96.0	
Total		560	100.1*	420	100.1*	8.45 (< 0.01)
Change in bowel or bladder habits	Yes	51	18.7	81	11.5	
	No	222	81.3	626	88.5	
Total		273	100.0	707	100.0	8.82 (< 0.01)
Difficulty swallowing	Yes	6	7.1	37	4.1	
	No	79	92.9	858	95.9	
Total		85	100.0	895	100.0	1.58 (NS)
Change in a wart or mole	Yes	29	9.5	46	6.8	
	No	276	90.5	629	93.2	
Total		305	100.0	675	100.0	2.16 (NS)
Persistent cough	Yes	260	55.1	243	47.8	
	No	212	44.9	265	52.2	
Total		472	100.0	508	100.0	5.15 (< 0.05)

*Total differs from 100 percent due to rounding errors.

stated one or two of the seven, whereas 66 percent of the callers compared to 51 percent of the controls were able to state correctly three or more.

These data carry several implications, especially when we compare them with the data reported in Table 7.7. First, the presence of possible cancer-related problems tended to increase the proportion of both callers and controls who were able to mention three or more danger signals correctly. This lends support to our hypothesis that presence of cancer-related problems increases awareness of health matters, especially cancer. Second, differences between callers and controls also increase when callers with cancer symptoms are compared to controls with cancer symptoms and when these differences are compared to the basic caller-control differences in Table 7.7. For instance, a 16 percent difference was found when cancer symptoms were present as opposed to only an 8 percent difference when all callers and controls interviewed were compared. Thus, the presence of possible cancer-related problems did seem to affect knowledge. On the other hand, this may be viewed as a result of contact with the program. However, once again, we must qualify this conclusion since callers still may have been more knowledgeable than controls before contacting the program.

Another way to investigate the degree of knowledge obtained from contact with the program is to group the topics listened to with respect to their appropriate danger signals, then to cross-tabulate responses concerning those seven signals with the tape heard (Table 7.11). We would hypothesize that those individuals who listened to a particular subject would be more likely to give the relevant danger signal correctly than those who listened to other topics. With the exception of topics concerning sores that do not heal, we do find a tendency for callers who listened to a particular topic to be more likely to state the appropriate warning signal correctly than those who did not listen to that subject. The differences, although statistically significant, tend to be small. However, when we group all of the topics together in the manner of Table 7.12, we once again find statistically significant differences although the overall difference remains about 7 percent. These data show a small but consistent tendency for callers who have listened to a particular topic to be somewhat more likely to cite correctly the appropriate warning signal.

Finally, another measure of impact may be made by comparing the importance of a particular cancer site with the popularity of that topic. In Table 7.13, we have rank ordered the cancer incidence for the most frequent sites in the United States by sex (Levin et al. 1974). For purposes of comparison, we have also rank ordered the Can-Dial response according to topic by sex. As can be seen from Table 7.13, Can-Dial response tended to approximate the importance of

Table 7.12 Topic Selected and Response to the Appropriate
            Danger Signal

Selected	Correct		Incorrect	
	Number	Percent	Number	Percent
Yes	511	18.3	469	11.6
No	2,289	81.7	3,590	88.4
Total	2,800	100.0	4,059	100.0

Note: $\chi^2 = 60.65$, P < 0.001, 1 df

the appropriate site. For instance, among males, lung cancer comprises the site of highest incidence. Correspondingly, the most popular male topic was "If You Want to Give up Cigarettes," followed
by "The Effect of Cigarette Smoking on Non-Smokers," and "Lung
Cancer" not far below that. Cancer of the prostate, however, which
ranks number two for males, occurred further down the list. Since
this is primarily a cancer of old age, and since elderly males made
poor use of the Can-Dial program, this finding is probably not unfore-
seen. Colo-rectal cancer, which is also a significant male problem,
was a more popular subject. Bladder and gastric cancer do not appear
on the rank ordering of male selections. Popularity of cancer of the
breast as a topic is interesting since it is a rare male site. However,
it could be a result of interest and concern shown by male spouses.
For females, we find a somewhat closer relationship between topics
selected and importance of site. Breast cancer, which is the number-
one female site, was the second most popular topic requested.
Cigarette-related subjects ranked first, fifth, and seventh for females.*
This may reflect concern on the part of women for spouses who smoke
or about the smoking problem in general in that more women are now
smoking. Colo-rectal cancer and topics concerning uterine cancer
and the Pap test were also frequently requested by females. Although
the correspondence is not perfect, these data do tend to show that
information regarding the most common sites was requested by callers and consequently found its way out to the public. This also can
be viewed as evidence of the program's value.

---

*Lung cancer has been rapidly increasing among women. If the
trend continues, lung cancer will soon exceed breast cancer.

Table 7.13 Cancer Incidence and Response to Can-Dial

U.S. Cancer Incidence by Site and Sex, 1969-1971		Response to Can-Dial by Site and Sex	
R/O Male Cancer	R/O Female Cancer	R/O Male Response	R/O Female Response
1. Lung and bronchus	Breast	1. If You Want to Give up Cigarettes	If You Want to Give up Cigarettes
2. Prostate	Colo-rectal	2. Cancer's Warning Signals	Cancer of the Breast
3. Colo-rectal	Cervix (in situ)	3. Effects of Cigarette Smoking on Non-Smokers	Cancer of the Uterus
4. Bladder	Corpus uteri	4. What Is Cancer?	What Are Cancer's Warning Signals?
5. Stomach	Cervix (invasive)	5. Lung Cancer	Effects of Cigarette Smoking on Non-Smokers
6. Total leukemia	Lung and bronchus	6. Cancer of the Breast	Cancer of the Colon and Rectum
7. Pancreas	Ovary	7. Cancer of the Skin	What Is Cancer?
8. Lymphoma	Lymphoma	8. Cancer of the Colon and Rectum	Cigarette Smoking and the Pregnant Woman
9. Larynx	Pancreas	9. Cancer of the Brain	What Is the Pap Test?
10. Kidney	Total leukemia	10. Leukemia	Cancer of the Skin
		11. Cancer of the Prostate	Leukemia
		12. Hodgkin's Disease	Lung Cancer
		13. Cancer of the Mouth	Hodgkin's Disease

CONCLUSION

In this chapter, we have examined the evidence concerning the possible impact of Can-Dial upon users. We have seen that approximately 40 percent of the respondents interviewed reported taking some type of health-related action. We have also seen that the presence of health problems in general did not seem to exert any significant influence upon callers with regard to behavior change. A large percentage of Can-Dial users reported talking to someone about the information they received from the program, and a substantial percentage of those with whom the information was discussed also took some form of relevant action. Concerning knowledge, we have seen that callers tended to be able to mention correctly and in a consistent manner more of the seven danger signals than noncaller controls. When cases with and without problems were examined, once again we found that the presence of problems made little or no difference to knowledge. However, when cases with possible cancer symptoms were compared to controls with such symptoms, we found that cases correctly cited more of the seven danger signals than controls. We also found some correlation between listening to a topic and subsequently being able to mention correctly the appropriate warning signal. Finally, a correspondence was found between important cancer sites and requests from the public for tapes concerning these sites.

8

PROMOTION AND RESPONSE

Throughout the three-year program, Can-Dial was extensively publicized in the Erie County area. Advertising took place through several means. Most of the promotional efforts relied upon public service time and space obtained from local television stations, radio stations, newspapers, and other types of community publications. Brochures were also developed that offered the telephone number and listed the topics available. These were distributed through various means such as by mail and in supermarkets, places of business, libraries, schools, physicians' offices, dentists' offices, hospitals, and churches. Records were kept of the amount and type of promotional activity engaged in, as well as of location.

Figure 8.1 illustrates the total number of calls received, the number of brochures distributed, and the number of television and radio announcements that occurred for the three-year period. Erie County response was highest during the first year of Can-Dial's operation and decreased by about 5,000 calls a year for each of the following two years. With regard to amounts of promotion, the greatest number of pamphlets were distributed during the first year, followed by years three and two in that order. Television and radio announcements were largely beyond our control since the times when these were aired were at the discretion of the stations involved. However, more of these occurred during Can-Dial's first year than in the two later years. Missing from this breakdown is the effect upon response of other forms of media such as newspapers and the classified pages telephone White Directory. However, it is difficult to document these items in terms of amounts since newspapers are distributed throughout the Erie County area and we were not given notice of when advertisements would appear. Furthermore, the

Figure 8.1 Response and Major Forms of Promotion

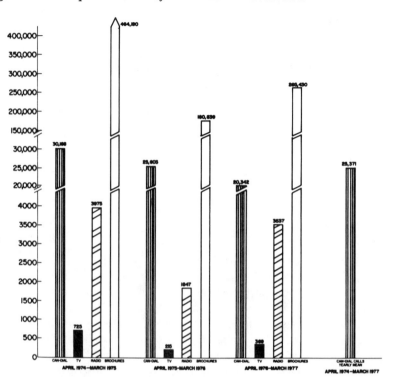

telephone classified pages White Directory was distributed every year
to all telephone subscribers. Consequently, these data should be
viewed in conjunction with material presented in Chapter 3 concerning
source of information, especially Table 3.4. It will be recalled that
television and radio, as information sources, accounted for approximately 13 percent of the response; newspapers about 6 percent; pamphlets (including all forms and places of distribution) about 36 percent; and classified telephone directory about 30 percent. Sixty-four
percent of the calls cited sources that were free of cost to the Can-
Dial program, brochures being the only type of promotion that
incurred costs.

Figures 8.2, 8.3, and 8.4 compare the calls received and the
major types of promotion distributed for each month during the three-
year period. For the purposes of comparison, we have presented
these as line graphs although they are more properly viewed as histograms. It is difficult to relate response with type of promotion pre-
cisely. There is some indication of a relationship between calls
received and the number of pamphlets distributed from April 1974
through March 1975. A decrease in calls received each year during
the late winter and spring months through early summer is noticeable.

Figure 8.2 Calls Received and Promotion, April 1974—March 1975

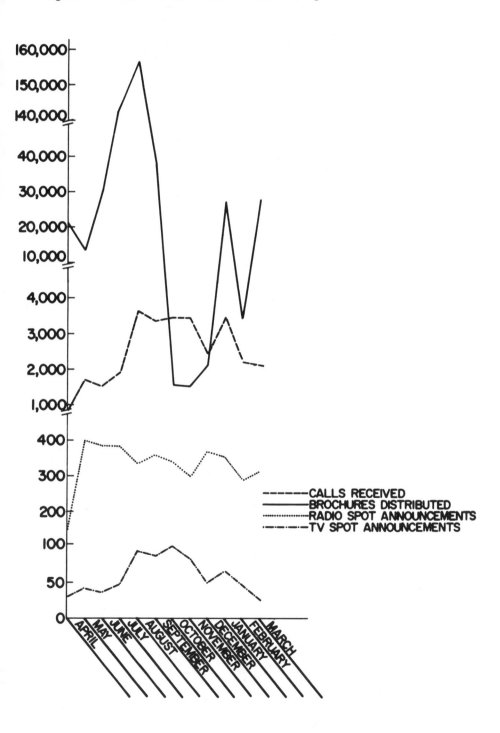

Figure 8.3 Calls Received and Promotion, April 1975—March 1976

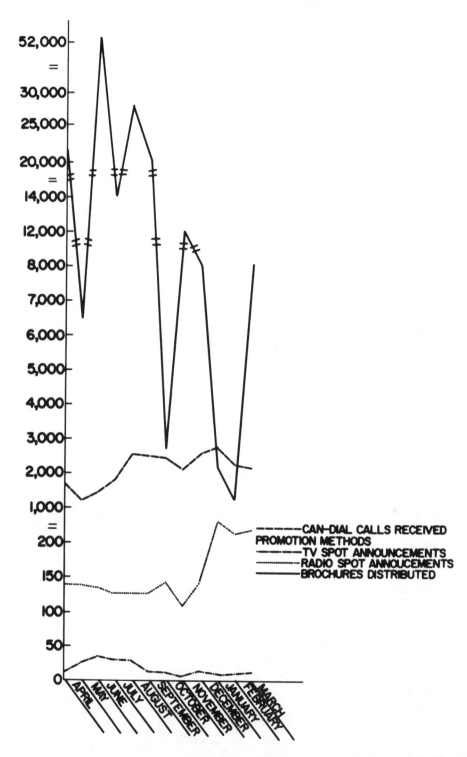

Figure 8.4 Calls Received and Promotion, April 1976—March 1977

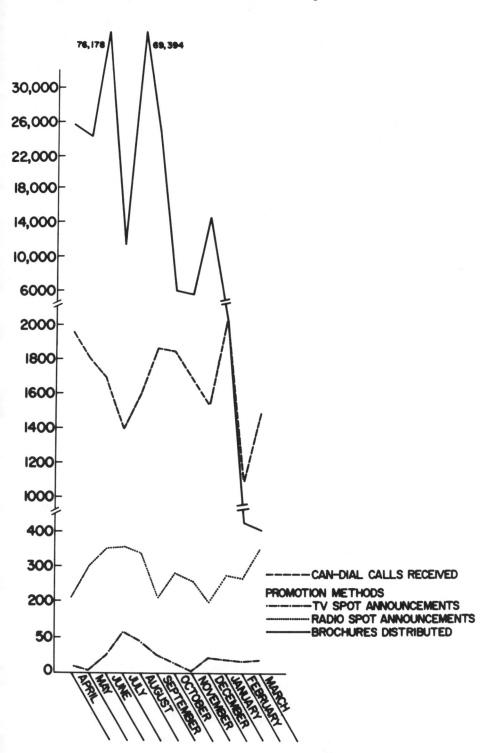

The slight upturn seen during 1976 probably resulted from national publicity given to the effects of radiation upon thyroid cancer. Response during the early summer of 1976 was low in comparison to previous years. Although promotional activities may have had a general effect upon response, this is not easily observed through crude measures.

Similar findings were observed when the number of calls received each month was compared to the number of brochures distributed and the number of television and radio announcements made. One would hypothesize that periods of high promotional activity would be reflected in high levels of use. This was not the case. In fact, we were unable to detect significant relationships between use and the amount of promotion by month and by quarter for each year.

Undoubtedly, promotional activities do have an effect on response, as will be shown later in this chapter. However, comparison of the proportion of calls received with the proportional distribution of three major forms of advertising of the system does not show a strong effect during each time period examined.

Early in the program, we became aware of an increase in calls immediately after a public service announcement had been aired over television. Figures 8.5-8.10 show the relationship between the times of the television announcements and calls received. As is illustrated in these figures, we were able to link some of the peaks in response to times when advertisements were aired, although it was not possible to identify all television and radio announcements. Once again, one should keep in mind that these are more properly viewed as histograms and do not comprise continuous functions since calls were grouped by hour. These data show that an increase in calls occurred immediately following a television announcement, but this increase did not continue very long. In all probability, if interested individuals who were watching were unable to reach the operator immediately because lines were busy, they either forgot the phone number or lost interest in calling. Television advertisements may be effective, as is demonstrated by these data, but they are so only for short periods of time. Much of their effectiveness probably depends upon the times during which they take place. When we examined this aspect, we found they were often aired during the early hours of the morning when few people would be watching television and when the Can-Dial service was not in operation. Another way of determining the relationship between Can-Dial use and television advertisements would be to compare observed with expected use during a defined period of time. Figures 8.11, 8.12, and 8.13 show the proportional distribution of calls during one year's operation by hour compared to the proportional response for defined days. Although we were unable to correlate all of the peaks that occurred with specific announcements, we

Figure 8.5 Television Announcements and Hourly Response,
            May 2, 1974

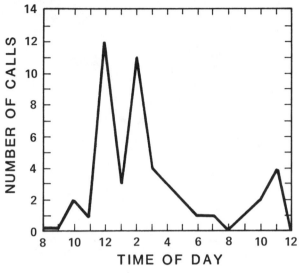

TELEVISION STATION	TIME OF ANNOUNCEMENT
CH. 7	6:53 AM
CH. 7	11:18 AM
CH. 2	1:27 PM

Figure 8.6 Television Announcements and Hourly Response,
            May 24, 1974

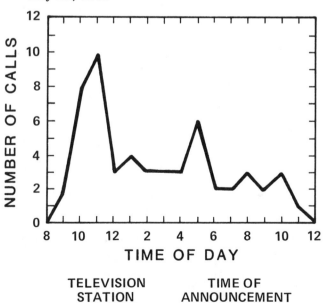

TELEVISION STATION	TIME OF ANNOUNCEMENT
CH. 2	9:27 AM
CH. 7	9:33 AM

Figure 8.7 Television Announcements and Hourly Response,
           July 10, 1974

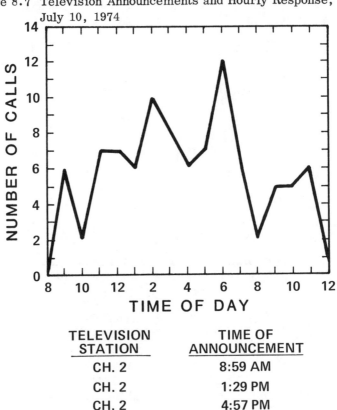

TELEVISION	TIME OF
STATION	ANNOUNCEMENT
CH. 2	8:59 AM
CH. 2	1:29 PM
CH. 2	4:57 PM

Figure 8.8 Television Announcements and Hourly Response,
           December 29, 1975

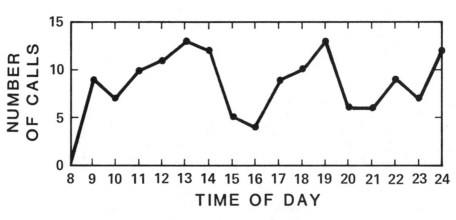

TELEVISION	TIME OF
STATION	ANNOUNCEMENT
CH. 7	11:28 AM
CH. 7	11:24 PM

Figure 8.9 Television Announcements and Hourly Response,
July 19, 1976

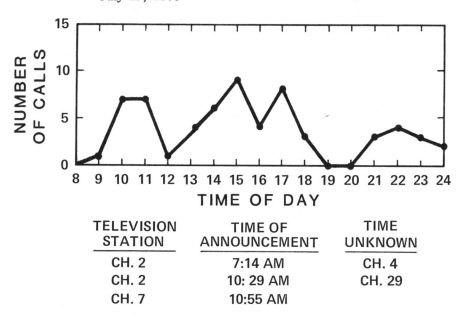

TELEVISION STATION	TIME OF ANNOUNCEMENT	TIME UNKNOWN
CH. 2	7:14 AM	CH. 4
CH. 2	10: 29 AM	CH. 29
CH. 7	10:55 AM	

Figure 8.10 Television Announcements and Hourly Response,
August 11, 1976

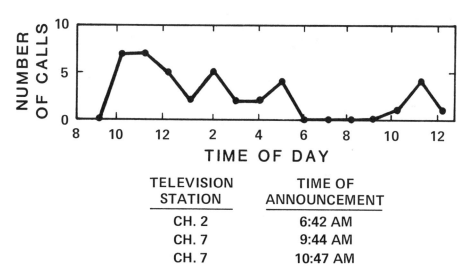

TELEVISION STATION	TIME OF ANNOUNCEMENT
CH. 2	6:42 AM
CH. 7	9:44 AM
CH. 7	10:47 AM

Figure 8.11 Observed and Expected Response, December 24, 1975
and April 1975–March 1976

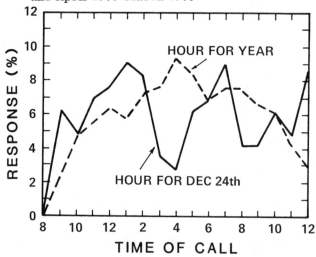

TV ANNOUNCEMENTS 11:28 AM, 11:24 PM

Figure 8.12 Observed and Expected Response, October 1, 1975
and April 1975–March 1976

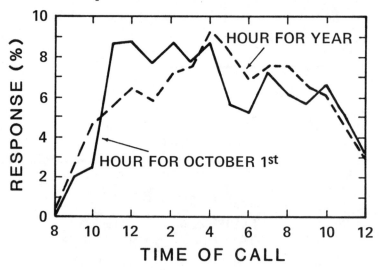

TV ANNOUNCEMENTS: 6.58 AM

Figure 8.13 Observed and Expected Response, February 9, 1976
and April 1975—March 1976

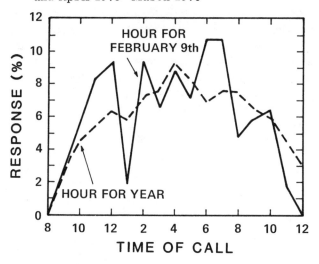

TV ANNOUNCEMENT: SOMETIME IN AM

Figure 8.14 Promotion and Response in Selected Towns

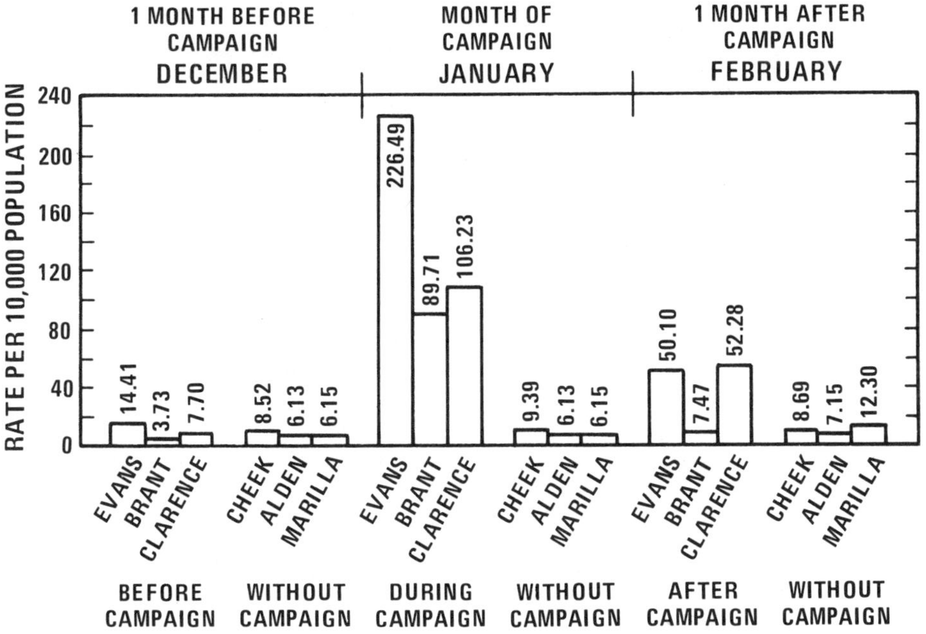

Source: G. S. Wilkinson, E. A. Mirand, and S. Graham,
"Measuring Response to a Cancer Information Telephone Facility:
Can-Dial," American Journal of Public Health 66, no. 4 (1976):
367-71. Reprinted with permission of the American Public Health
Association.

were able to do it often enough to demonstrate that they did have an effect upon response. For instance, in Figure 8.11 we can see that announcements occurred at 11:29 A.M. and 11:24 P.M. Immediately after these, an increase in calls occurred greater than that expected based on one year's experience.

After we became aware of low response in certain areas of Erie County, we conducted experiments to see if use could be increased through additional promotional activities. Figure 8.14 shows the results of a promotional campaign conducted in three townships compared to three control townships in which no promotional activ-

Table 8.1 Response and Promotional Mailings in Selected Cities and Towns

		Monthly Response	Percent Monthly Response for 3-Month Period	Total 3-Month Response for Each Town
Lackawanna	Before	35	5.8	
	During	142	23.6	601
	After	24	4.0	
Grand Island	Before	10	2.4	
	During	122	29.7	411
	After	24	5.8	
Williamsville	Before	36	7.9	
	During	60	13.2	454
	After	36	7.9	
Tonawanda	Before	139	14.9	
	During	114	12.2	935
	After	70	7.5	
Depew	Before	40	10.6	
	During	67	17.7	379
	After	42	11.1	
Clarence	Before	20	8.9	
	During	35	15.6	225
	After	19	8.4	
Evans	Before	21	4.0	
	During	58	11.0	525
	After	80	15.2	

Source: G. S. Wilkinson, E. A. Mirand, and S. Graham, Cancer Information by Telephone: A Two-Year Evaluation, Health Education Monographs, vol. 5, no. 3, pp. 251-65, 1977. Reprinted with permission of the Society for Public Health Education, Inc.

ities took place. During the month of the campaign, the number of calls from the three experimental townships increased dramatically compared to response the month before and to response from the three control townships. Calls from these three towns remained higher one month after the campaign than it had been one month before it, and this indicated a continuation of increased interest. By comparison, response in the three control towns showed little or no difference during this three-month period. These results demonstrate that response from low utilizing areas can be increased by increasing promotional activities there.

Similar experiments were continued for a time in the form of brochures mailed directly to residences in selected areas. Table 8.1 shows that in almost every case the monthly response increased substantially during and sometimes after the mailings. Once again, use of the system was increased by means of increased promotional activities. However, brochures are costly to distribute since they involve mailing as well as printing costs.

It is interesting that, when small studies or experiments involving promotion were undertaken, we were able to see the effect that increased promotional activities had upon calls received. However, we have not been able to demonstrate in any noticeable manner the link between overall Can-Dial response and promotional activities in general. Although there is some evidence that calls were frequent during periods of high promotional activity, enough ambiguity is involved to preclude arriving at definite conclusions. In all probability, response is affected by a large variety of factors, including news items such as the death of a prominent individual from cancer or new developments in cancer research or treatment.

9

CONCLUSIONS
AND RECOMMENDATIONS

All too often, educational and other health service programs are offered with either no or inadequate attempts at evaluation. The Can-Dial program was conceived essentially as an experiment involving, on the one hand, operation of a dial-access cancer information system and, on the other hand, investigation of ways of eliciting community response and evaluating factors effecting this response, as well as of the efficacy of such an approach. In this document, we have attempted to describe the system and present findings resulting from three years of evaluation of the program.

Can-Dial was a dial-access system consisting of 51 pre-recorded taped presentations, 4 telephone lines, and an automatic playback console manned by an operator 16 hours a day, 7 days a week. Upon contacting the program, callers requested a topic from the operator, who inserted the tape cassette and activated the playback mechanism. Presentations varied from one to seven minutes in length. Subject matter included cancer research, cancer etiology, clinical features, symptoms, action to be taken if symptoms are encountered, modes of management and prevention, and other information whenever relevant.

Continuous monitoring of calls showed variations in patterns of response that can be used for future planning or the development of similar systems by others. These include variations in hourly and daily response that showed the afternoon and work week to be most productive of calls. About 60 percent of the calls were by individuals who had not previously used the system, and 17 percent were repeat calls. Brochures stimulated over half of the response, and public service announcements over the local media generated about 30 percent. Increased distribution of brochures in several experimental

communities usually resulted in increased use for a short period of
time. Although they incur printing and sometimes mailing costs,
brochures obviously work. In fact, forms of promotion that provide
the phone number and topics appear to be the most effective.

Analyses of user characteristics show that: about twice as
many females as males responded; use was highest among teenagers
and steadily declined with increasing age; students and housewives
were the most frequent users when occupation was considered; and
response declined with increasing distance of residence from the
institute's downtown location. Although a small tendency was observed
for upper SES groups to use the program more than lower status
groups, a more important difference was that between rural residents
and those in the city and suburbs.

Telephone interviews of over 1,000 callers, conducted some
weeks after the call, showed that most were motivated to use the program because they wanted to quit smoking or had experienced some
kind of contact with cancer or other illness in themselves, family, or
friends. Approximately 40 percent of the respondents reported taking
health-related action as a result of contacting the program, and
another 40 percent reported no change in behavior. A significant portion of the callers reported talking about the information to others,
with about 12 percent of these others visiting a physician or clinic.
Finally, comparison of callers with a like sample of noncaller controls demonstrated that callers were able to cite correctly more
danger signals than were noncallers.

In comparing callers with noncallers, the demographic differences that we found suggest that callers were more likely to be
younger and better educated than noncallers, whereas noncallers
were more often retired or widowed than callers. These are similar
to other findings showing adoption to be greater among younger and
more educated individuals (Janni et al. 1960; Winkelstein and Graham
1959). They also complement our earlier findings showing older
groups making less use of the system than younger groups (Wilkinson
et al. 1976b; 1977b). This lower response cannot be attributed to a
lack of time or access since the widowed, retired, and elderly are
more likely to have adequate time for contacting a program such as
Can-Dial than are younger people who are working. We suggest that
one's orientation toward health may be reflected in these demographic
differences: younger people are more open to stimuli by media, they
are more prevention-oriented and perhaps more optimistic about
health, whereas older people are more treatment-oriented and perhaps
more fatalistic. Higher levels of education may exert a favorable
influence in that increased schooling may lead to increased use of
preventive health services. As expected, callers were more likely
than controls to have had some kind of close contact with cancer

patients, especially among family members. The lower use by widows may reflect less exposure to important sources of information from within the family. On the other hand, general contact with the health care system, whether through employment in one of the health professions or through personal illness experience, did not seem to exert a significant influence. The presence of health problems or symptoms that might arouse one's concern about cancer, however, does seem important for prompting some individuals to contact the program. This finding is important for several reasons. It demonstrates that more individuals who might benefit from early diagnosis and possibly treatment use the program than others. It also supports our expectation that a cancer information facility would be of greater interest to individuals who suspected they might have cancer than those who did not. Finally, these data agree with suggestions by other investigators that such facilities must be compatible with the expectations and experiences of target populations if these populations are to make use of the innovation in question (see Yeracaris 1961; Ellenbogen and Lowe 1968; Becker and Maiman 1975).

That more callers who contacted the program than controls were smokers also would support these contentions as well as suggest that a portion of the smoking public is perhaps becoming more willing to try to stop smoking. It is possible to speculate that warnings regarding the hazards of smoking are at least raising the concern of susceptible individuals. Previous studies have suggested that early users are sometimes more likely to rely upon printed media whereas later users rely upon electronic media (Graham 1973). Our results indicate that callers were more likely to be users of electronic media, at least in terms of regularly watching more television stations, whereas noncallers displayed some tendency toward more variety in newspaper consumption. Frequency of using television, radio, newspapers, and magazines revealed no interesting differences. However, when we compared callers with possible cancer symptoms to controls with such symptoms, differences in frequency of use of television and radio did begin to assume some importance. Most investigators have reported that mass media are used more among higher than lower social classes and that users are likely to become aware of innovations through the mass media (Heagarty et al. 1968; Pope et al. 1971). Our findings seem to suggest that variety in media use is more important than amount per se. We did not find callers to use the mass media more than controls.

The ability of callers to list correctly more of the seven danger signals may demonstrate retention of knowledge received as a result of using the program, assuming both callers and controls have been exposed to similar amounts of information from sources such as the American Cancer Society. Similar findings have been reported for an

American Cancer Society study that used leaflets describing the seven warning signals. Our results are also similar regarding signals frequently mentioned correctly, such as the presence of lumps, unusual bleeding, and sores that do not heal, and those rarely mentioned, including changes in bowel habits and difficulty swallowing. Additional education pertaining to the latter appears warranted. As expected, we found callers to display a greater orientation toward preventive health care through regular Pap tests, breast self-examination, routine checkups, and being more likely to have recently suggested to someone that he or she see a physician. Thus dial-access systems are somewhat more likely to appeal to those who are already prevention-minded. These findings compare favorably with those suggesting that a service be compatible with one's value orientation. However, we still need to discover ways to reach those who are not oriented toward preventive health care.

Several limitations of cancer information services such as Can-Dial are suggested by these findings. The widowed, elderly, and less educated have to be approached through different means, as do males in general. Increased efforts are required to make people more aware of the benefits of a preventive health orientation compared to a problem orientation. Obvious starting points as channels for dissemination of such information are existing educational facilities, places of work, and organizations catering to older people, as well as hospitals and physicians' offices. It should be remembered that dial-access systems complement rather than supplant the educational functions of health professionals. Concern demonstrated by smokers suggests that continued and perhaps even increased activity in the area of smoking clinics and other smoking dissuasion efforts are needed. Finally, information in the printed media, such as question-and-answer columns, short informative articles, and perhaps even regular syndicated columns, might appeal to that portion of the public more predisposed to written than electronic media.

Our findings have implications for those who would enhance public knowledge and improve behavior oriented toward control of cancer. For example, we have demonstrated the continued difficulty of making the program useful to those at high risk: males and older people. As has been found elsewhere, rural residents used it less than others. Our experiments in various communities throughout Erie County, however, suggest that utilization can be increased substantially through the direct mailing of a brochure that describes the program and furnishes the phone number. Direct mail is a simple and direct approach. It is possible that more elaborate measures would be even more effective.

It is interesting that the frequency with which various topics are requested reflects to some extent the magnitude of risk of the cancer in question. Thus, the most frequently requested topics have dealt with frequently occurring types such as cancer of the lung, breast, cervix, colon, and rectum. The substantial percentage of requests for information on lung cancer and ways to stop smoking implied a need that the public felt and that public health activities were not meeting. About one-quarter of the callers asserted that they reduced or quit smoking after listening to the Can-Dial tapes. We have no way of knowing the part played by the tapes in this action. It is likely that many already had decided to stop and merely called Can-Dial to obtain reinforcement of their decision. Nevertheless, tobacco is one of the most important pathogens in industrial societies today; it is related etiologically to a number of diseases, and inexpensive public health measures that can play a part in reducing smoking are much to be desired.

Our reservations continue regarding the role of Can-Dial in bringing about the various new behaviors reported by respondents after listening to tapes. It is necessary to inquire further, perhaps in personal interviews, as to the factors affecting decisions resulting in different types of behavior. At this moment we can say little more than that callers appeared to take steps that could control cancer after they had called. Moreover, a fair number of those with whom callers discussed information obtained from Can-Dial took desired action such as consulting a physician.

We suspect that Can-Dial may have functioned as one facet of a congeries of stimuli that preceded taking cancer control behavior. The fact that callers knew more of cancer's danger signals indicates the likely importance of the American Cancer Society's long-term activities. We suspect that discussions with friends and physicians, acquaintance with cancer in friends and family members, plus Can-Dial, when taken together all played a part in any behavior change undertaken. Possibly, a dial-access system can figure as an adjunct to other, more conventional health education efforts in the future. We do not feel that dial-access systems alone can by themselves bring about long-term behavior change of a significant nature in significant segments of the population. Other approaches are needed to complement the Can-Dial approach.

All of this assumes that the telephone information system used is similar to Roswell Park Memorial Institute's Can-Dial and that the public health agency utilizing it has the resources available: approximately $1.56 per call, including cost of brochures and their distribution. We found that peak times of calling were midweek and midday, which means that sufficient numbers of operators, telephone lines, and tapes must be available at those times so as not to discourage would-be audiences. The mechanics of operation have been described. Our experiments suggest that publicizing the availability of the facility can increase its use greatly; this should accompany inauguration of the system. In light of the meager state of our knowledge regarding the ways, if any, in which such facilities can enhance knowledge and behavior change for the control of cancer, we need new inquiries into the subject.

It would appear that telephone health education systems may be effective and that they may be used more in the future. They can serve to answer many of the users' pressing questions in privacy at a time and place of their choosing and at no cost to them. From the health educator's point of view, unlike many audiences, the caller is self-selected to be interested in the subject and to pay special heed to the information provided. Our evidence suggests that he or she may even take some desired actions partly as a result of the call. Clearly, however, more research to evaluate such facilities is necessary to establish their mode of operation and their worth.

Other types of evidence of Can-Dial's value also exist. For instance, the program provided practical answers to practical questions often raised by the public concerning such matters as how to stop smoking, how to do breast self-examination, and what the Pap test is and where it is obtained. It has already been noted that subjects were requested by callers in approximate proportion to their importance in terms of incidence. If programs such as Can-Dial did not exist, one might ask where or of whom the public would ask such questions. Many do not have access to medical textbooks, and physicians often do not have time to answer such questions. There is a functional need for this type of information that Can-Dial fulfilled. This comprises a commonsense measure of the value of such programs.

Additional clues to the system's value include indicators of user satisfaction such as solicited and unsolicited comments from callers, which have been overwhelmingly favorable. The large number of repeat calls may demonstrate that callers found their first contact worthwhile. Many requests for information about the system have been received from private individuals and organizations from around the world. Finally, the large number of calls received by the program during its initial three years of existence shows that a large segment of the populace perceives a need for cancer information and will respond to the dial-access method.*

---

*Those who currently administer the Can-Dial system report that a similar volume of calls is still received, although the service has been expanded to cover all of New York State. This is especially remarkable in light of the fact that Can-Dial has now been in operation for almost a decade!

Dial-access information systems serve a useful purpose. They can be used to provide basic information to the general public cheaply, quickly, and relatively effectively. They seem to attract individuals who have been exposed to problems in that general area—in this case, those who were knowledgeable about cancer, oriented toward preventive medicine, and somewhat more conversationally inclined. Ancillary methods designed to reach nonutilizing segments of the population identified in this report need to be designed. Evaluation of these alternative methods should be incorporated into their design and initial operation. Publicizing efforts appear to be transitory and must be continued. At the same time, new approaches need to be developed. Finally, dial-access facilities must be complemented by well-designed alternative education and health programs that reinforce behaviors that may have been stimulated.

Appendix A

Caller Code Sheet

CALLER CODE SHEET

Card 1

	CALLER NUMBER						LINE		DATE OF CALL					TIME				REQ.	
1	2	3	4	5	6	7	8	9	10	11	12	13	14	15	16	17	18	19	20
1																	■		

TAPES		TYPE		SOURCE				LAST NAME											
21	22	23	24	25	26	27	28	29	30	31	32	33	34	35	36	37	38	39	40
		■		■			■												

INITIAL		STREET NUMBER						STREET NAME											
41	42	43	44	45	46	47	48	49	50	51	52	53	54	55	56	57	58	59	60
■		■																	■

				CITY								STATE				ZIP			
61	62	63	64	65	66	67	68	69	70	71	72	73	74	75	76	77	78	79	80

Card 2

	CALLER NUMBER						COUNTY			TELEPHONE							AGE		
1	2	3	4	5	6	7	8	9	10	11	12	13	14	15	16	17	18	19	20
2						■			■								■		

SEX		OCCUPATION																	
21	22	23	24	25	26	27	28	29	30	31	32	33	34	35	36	37	38	39	40
■		■																	

41	42	43	44	45	46	47	48	49	50	51	52	53	54	55	56	57	58	59	60

61	62	63	64	65	66	67	68	69	70	71	72	73	74	75	76	77	78	79	80

Appendix B

Interview Schedules

INTERVIEW SCHEDULES

OMB 68 S74107
Exp. 4/1977

Roswell Park Memorial Institute
Can-Dial Evaluation of Callers
February 1975

This is _____ from Roswell Park
Memorial Institute. Recently you called our Can-Dial program. We
would like to get some idea as to how this project is working so that
we can make improvements that might be needed. We would like
your reaction to the tape you heard and would like to ask you some
questions about health care in general. Do you have a few moments?
(Only if needed: "Your replies will be kept completely confidential.")

Name _____ Date _____ Age _____

Address _____ City or Town _____

C.T. _____ Tape Number and Subject _____

Date Contacted Can-Dial _____ Sex: Male ___ Female ___

Can-Dial Caller Number _____ Telephone # _____

1. Where did you first hear about Can-Dial? _____

_____

	Date	Time	Channel/Station/Name
Television			
Radio			
Newspaper			
Brochure (Obtained where?)			
Other (List)			

2. Why did you call Can-Dial? _____

_____

_____

3. Were your questions answered, or did you have still more ques-
    tions after listening to the tape?

    > Yes, questions answered _____
    > No, still more questions _____

    a. If no, what types of questions? _____
    _____
    _____

4. Are there any services you would like to see added? _____
    _____
    _____

5. What did you do as a result of hearing the tape? _____
    _____

6. Did you talk to anyone about the information you obtained from
    the tapes? Yes ____ No ____

    If yes:

    a. Whom did you talk to? _____

    b. What did you talk about? _____

    c. Did he/she visit an M.D. or clinic? _____

7. Whom do you usually talk to about health matters? _____

8. Do you know anyone personally who has cancer now or who had
    it in the past?   Yes ____ No ____

    a. If yes, who? What type of cancer?

Spouse	__	_____	Brother	__	_____
Father	__	_____	Sister	__	_____
(in-law)	__	_____	Aunt	__	_____
Mother	__	_____	Uncle	__	_____
(in-law)	__	_____	Friend	__	_____
Child	__	_____	Acquaintance	__	_____
Grandparent	__	_____			
Cousin	__	_____			

9. Do you have any friends or relatives who work in one of the
    health fields?

    Yes ____   No ____

If yes:

a.   Relationship   b.   Type of job

Spouse   _____   1.   Physician _____
Child   _____   2.   Nurse   _____
Parent   _____   3.   Orderly   _____
Grandparent   _____   4.   Aide   _____
Aunt/uncle   _____   5.   Dietician _____
Cousin   _____   6.   Other   _____
Friend   _____
Brother   _____
Sister   _____

10.   In general, how is your health now? _____
      _____

11.   Do you have any health problems?   Yes ____   No ____

      If yes:

      a.   Describe _____
           _____

      b.   Have you seen a doctor about it/them?   Yes ___ No ___

      c.   Have you been in a hospital about it/them? Yes ___ No ___

12.   Have you visited a doctor during the past year? Yes ___ No ___

      a.   If yes, how many times? _____

      b.   How many times when you were not sick, such as for rou-
           tine checkups, shots, etc? _____

      c.   Have you told any friends or relatives to see a doctor in
           the past year?   Yes ____   No ____

      d.   If yes, why? _____

13.   Did you ever smoke?   Yes ____   No ____

      a.   Have you stopped?   Yes ____   No ____

      b.   If yes, why? _____

                      FEMALE RESPONDENTS ONLY

14.   Have you ever heard of the Pap test?   Yes ____   No ____

If yes:

   a.   Have you had one?   Yes ____   No ____

   b.   How often do you usually have one? _____

15.   Have you ever heard of the breast self exam? Yes ___   No ___

   If yes:

   a.   Do you give yourself one?   Yes ____   No ____

   b.   How often? _____

MALES & FEMALES

16.   How often do you get a chest X-ray? _____

17.   Are you married?   Yes ____   No ____

   a.   If no, are you separated ____ divorced ____ widowed __

      or never married? ____ (check one)

   b.   Do you have any children at home? Yes ____   No ____

   If yes:

   c.   How many? _____   d. What are their ages? _____

18.   Where were you born? _____

19.   How much schooling have you completed?

     1 2 3 4 5 6 7 8 9 10 11 12   1 2 3 4   4 plus

20.   What is the occupation of the head of your household? _____

21.   Do you watch television? Yes ____   No ____

   If yes:

   a.   What channels do you usually watch?

      2 __   4 __   7 __   9 __   11 __   12 __   17 __   29 __

      Others _____

   b.   Which hours? _____

22.   Do you listen to the radio?   Yes ____   No ____

If yes:

   a.   What stations do you usually listen to? _____

   b.   Which hours? _____

23.   Do you read any newspapers regularly? Yes _____ No _____

    If yes:

   a.   Which ones do you usually read? Courier Express _____

      Evening News _____ Other _____

   b.   How often? _____

24.   How often do you read articles by physicians in newspapers

    or magazines? Often_____ Rarely _____ Sometimes _____

   a.   If yes, which ones? (Name and list) _____

      _____

      _____

25.   Do you belong to any organizations, civic groups, etc.?
    Yes _____ No _____

26.   If yes, which ones? (Name and list) _____

    _____

27.   In your life, how many nights have you spent in a hospital?

    _____

28.   Can you tell me what the warning signals of cancer are? (List)

    _____   _____

    _____   _____

    _____   _____

    _____   _____

   a.   If a friend mentioned that he had one of these, what would

      you tell him to do? _____

      _____

   b.   If you yourself experienced one of these, what would you

      do? _____

      _____

THANK YOU FOR YOUR COOPERATION.

Interviewer _____

Interviewer's comments _____

_____

Coder _____   Code Checker _____

OMB 68 S74107
Exp. 4/1977

Roswell Park Memorial Institute
Can-Dial Evaluation of Controls

February 1975

This is _____ from the New York State Department of Health. We are conducting a health survey of Erie County residents to determine health care needs in the county. Your name was selected at random from the telephone directory. Do you have a few moments?

(Only if needed: "Your replies will be kept completely confidential.")

Name _____ Date _____ Age ____

Address _____ City or Town _____

C.T. _____ Code Number _____ Telephone # _____

Sex: Male ____ Female ____ Telephone Directory Page _____

1. Where were you born? _____

2. How much schooling have you completed?

   1 2 3 4 5 6 7 8 9 10 11 12   1 2 3 4   4 plus

3. What is your occupation? _____

4. What is the occupation of the head of your household? _____
   _____

5. Are you married?   Yes ____   No ____

   a. If no, are you separated ___ divorced ___ widowed ___ or
      never married? ___ (check one)

   b. Do you have any children at home?   Yes ____   No ____

   If yes:

   c. How many? _____   d. What are their ages? _____

6. In general, how is your health now? _____

7. Do you have any health problems?   Yes ____   No ____

   If yes:

   a. Describe _____

   _____

   b. Have you seen a doctor about it/them?   Yes ___ No ___

   c. Have you been in a hospital about it/them? Yes ___ No ___

FEMALE RESPONDENTS ONLY

8. Have you ever heard of the Pap test?   Yes ____   No ____

   If yes:

   a. Have you had one? Yes ____   No ____

   b. How often do you usually have one? _____

9. Have you ever heard of the breast self exam? Yes ____ No ___

   If yes:

   a. Do you give yourself one? Yes ____   No ____

   b. How often? _____

MALES AND FEMALES

10. How often do you get a chest X-ray? _____

11. Whom do you usually talk to about health matters? _____

12. Do you have any friends or relatives who work in one of the

    health fields?   Yes ____   No ____

    If yes:

    a. Relationship   b. Type of job

    Spouse   _____   1. Physician   _____
    Child   _____   2. Nurse   _____
    Parent   _____   3. Orderly   _____
    Grandparent _____   4. Aide   _____
    Aunt/uncle   _____   5. Dietician   _____
    Cousin   _____   6. Other   _____
    Friend   _____
    Brother   _____
    Sister   _____

13. Have you visited a doctor during the past year? Yes ___ No ___

    a. If yes, how many times? _____

    b. How many times when you were not sick, such as for routine checkups, shots, etc.? _____

    c. Have you told any friends or relatives to see a doctor in the past year? Yes ___ No ___

    d. If yes, why? _____

14. Did you ever smoke?   Yes ___   No ___

    a. Have you stopped?   Yes ___   No ___

    b. If yes, why? _____

15. Do you know anyone personally who has cancer now or who had it in the past?   Yes ___   No ___

    a. If yes, who? What type of cancer?

                           Type

Spouse	___ _____	Brother	___ _____
Father	___ _____	Sister	___ _____
(in-law)	___ _____	Aunt	___ _____
Mother	___ _____	Uncle	___ _____
(in-law)	___ _____	Friend	___ _____
Child	___ _____	Acquaintance	___ _____
Grandparent	___ _____		
Cousin	___ _____		

16. Do you watch television? Yes ___ No ___

    If yes:

    a. What channels do you usually watch?

       2 __ 4 __ 7 __ 9 __ 11 __ 12 __ 17 __ 29 __ Others __

    b. Which hours?

17. Do you listen to the radio? Yes ___ No ___

    If yes:

    a. What stations do you usually listen to? _____

    b. Which hours? _____

18. Do you read any newspapers regularly? Yes _____ No _____

    If yes:

    a. Which ones do you usually read? Courier Express _____

        Evening News _____   Other _____

    b. How often? _____

19. How often do you read articles by physicians in newspapers or

    magazines? Often _____   Rarely _____   Sometimes _____

    a. If yes, which ones? (Name and list) _____

        _____

20. Do you belong to any organizations, civic groups, etc.?
    Yes _____   No _____

21. a. If yes, which ones? (Name and list) _____

        _____

22. In your life, how many nights have you spent in a hospital? _____

23. Can you tell me what the warning signals of cancer are? (List)

    _____   _____

    _____   _____

    _____   _____

    _____   _____

    a. If a friend mentioned that he had one of these, what would

        you tell him to do? _____

        _____

    b. If you yourself experienced one of these, what would you do?

        _____

        _____

24. Have you ever heard of Can-Dial?   Yes _____   No _____

    If yes:

    a. How did you first hear about Can-Dial?

        Television   Brochure

        Radio   Friends or relatives

        Newspaper   Other

    b. Did you call Can-Dial?   Yes _____   No _____

25. Do you know anyone who has used Can-Dial? Yes ____ No __

    When? _____

    a.   If yes, for which subject? _____

26. Is there anything you would like to know about the Can-Dial

    program? _____

THANK YOU FOR YOUR COOPERATION.

Interviewer _____

Interviewer's comments _____

_____

Coder _____ Code Checker _____

BIBLIOGRAPHY

Bartlett, M. H., A. Johnston, and T. C. Meyer. 1973. "Dial Access Library Patient Information Service." New England Journal of Medicine, 288, pp. 994-98.

Becker, Marshall H., and L. A. Maiman. 1975. "Sociobehavioral Determinants of Compliance with Health and Medical Care Recommendations." Medical Care, 13, p. 10.

Doll, Richard, and Richard Peto. 1981. The Causes of Cancer. New York: Oxford University Press, pp. 1220-24.

Ellenbogen, B. L., and G. D. Lowe. 1968. "Health Care 'Styles' in Rural and Urban Areas." Rural Sociology, 33, p. 300.

Graham, Saxon. 1973. "Studies of Behavior Change to Enhance Public Health." American Journal of Public Health, 63, pp. 327-34.

Heagarty, Margaret C., Leon Robertson, John Kosa, and Joel J. Alpert. 1968. "Use of the Telephone by Low Income Families." Pediatrics, 73, pp. 740-44.

Hickey, R. C. 1971. "The Texas Regional Medical Program Dial Access Project for Cancer Consultation." Texas Medicine, 67, pp. 78-83.

Ianni, F. A., R. M. Albrecht, W. E. Bock, and A. K. Polan. 1960. "Age, Social, and Demographic Factors in Acceptance of Polio Vaccination." Public Health Reports, 75, pp. 545-56.

Levin, D. L., S. S. De Vesa, J. D. Godwin, and D. T. Silverman. 1974. Cancer Rates and Risks, 2nd ed. DHEW Pub. No. (NIH) 75-691. Washington, D.C.: U.S. Government Printing Office, p. 13.

Meyer, T. C., R. H. Hansen, R. T. Rogatz, and B. Mulvihill. 1970. "Providing Medical Information to Physicians by Telephone Tapes." Journal of Medical Information, 45, pp. 1060-65.

Pope, Clyde C., Samuel S. Yoshioka, and Merwyn R. Greenlick. 1971. "Determinants of Medical Care Utilization: The Use of the Telephone for Reporting Symptoms." Journal of Health and Social Behavior, 12, pp. 155-62.

Rens, Frank J., Diane M. Pinchoff, and James J. McCormack. 1974. County Data Source Book, vol. 1. Buffalo, N.Y.: Lakes Area Regional Medical Program.

U.S. Department of Commerce, Bureau of the Census. 1970. U.S. Census of the Population: 1970; Census Tract Statistics. Washington, D.C.: U.S. Government Printing Office.

Wilkinson, Gregg S. and John Wilson. 1983. "An Evaluation of Demographic Differences in the Utilization of a Cancer Information Service." Social Science and Medicine, 17, 3, pp. 169-75.

Wilkinson, Gregg S., Edwin A. Mirand, Debra L. Walsh, John L. Wilson, and Saxon Graham. 1978. "Utilization of a Cancer Telephone Information Facility: A Comparison of Callers and Non-Caller Controls." American Journal of Public Health, 68, pp. 1211-13.

Wilkinson, Gregg S., Edwin A. Mirand, Saxon Graham, Craig Johnson, and Joseph Vana. 1977a. "Can-Dial: A Dial Access Cancer Education Service." International Journal of Health Education, 20, pp. 158-63.

Wilkinson, Gregg S., Edwin A. Mirand, and Saxon Graham. 1977b. "Cancer Education by Telephone: A Two-Year Evaluation." Health Education Monographs, 5, pp. 251-63.

_____. 1976a. "Candial: An Experiment in Health Education and Cancer Control." Public Health Reports, 91, pp. 218-22.

_____. 1976b. "Measuring Response to a Cancer Information Telephone Facility." American Journal of Public Health, 66, pp. 367-71.

Winkelstein, Warren, and Saxon Graham. 1959. "Factors in Participation in the 1954 Poliomyelitis Vaccine Field Trials, Erie County, New York." American Journal of Public Health, 49, pp. 1454-66.

Yeracaris, Constantine A. 1961. "Social Factors Associated with the Acceptance of Medical Innovations: A Pilot Study." Journal of Health and Human Behavior, 3, pp. 193-98.

INDEX

ABOUT THE AUTHORS

SAXON GRAHAM is Professor and Chairman, Department of Social and Preventive Medicine, State University of New York at Buffalo, and Director of the Program in Social Epidemiology and the Control of Cancer. From 1966 until 1980 Dr. Graham was Professor, Department of Sociology, SUNY at Buffalo. Prior to 1966 he was Principal Cancer Research Scientist at Roswell Park Memorial Institute in Buffalo, New York.

Dr. Graham's research interests are in the areas of cancer epidemiology, health behavior, and cancer prevention through behavior change. He has published extensively in the areas of public health, cancer epidemiology, and behavior change. His articles have appeared in the American Journal of Epidemiology, Journal of the National Cancer Institute, Nutrition and Cancer, American Journal of Public Health, and numerous other professional journals.

Dr. Graham holds an A.B. from Amherst College, as well as an A.M. and Ph.D. from Yale University. He has also completed postgraduate work at the University of California at Berkeley and at the University of Buffalo.

EDWIN A. MIRAND is Associate Institute Director at Roswell Park Memorial Institute and Dean of the Roswell Park Memorial Institute Graduate Division of the State University of New York at Buffalo. His research activities are in the areas of experimental hematology, viral oncology, and gnotobiotics. He received a B.A. and M.A. from the State University of New York at Buffalo and a Ph.D. from the University of Syracuse. In addition, he is the recipient of two honorary Doctor of Science degrees awarded to him for his vigorous efforts in higher education. To name but two of his many citations, Dr. Mirand has been awarded the Billings Silver Medal by the American Medical Association and the award of the Medical Society of the State of New York for scientific research.

Among his many outside activities, Dr. Mirand is a Consultant to the National Institutes of Health, is past President and Director of the Association for Gnotobiotics, and is President of the International Society of Gnotobiology. He sits on the editorial boards of the Journal of Surgical Oncology and the Yearbook of Cancer. He is also Secretary-Treasurer of the Association of American Cancer Institutes, was Secretary General of the 13th International Cancer

Congress, and is Chairman of the USA National Committee/International Union Against Cancer, of the National Academy of Sciences.

GREGG S. WILKINSON is currently Group Leader of the Epidemiology Group, Health, Safety and Environment Divisiion at Los Alamos National Laboratory, University of California. He is also Associate Clinical Research Professor at the University of New Mexico School of Medicine in Albuquerque, New Mexico, and Associate Clinical Professor at the University of Colorado Medical Center in Denver, Colorado.

From 1978 to 1980 he was a Senior Epidemiologist with the Health Effects Research Laboratory, U. S. Environmental Protection Agency, Research Triangle Park, North Carolina. Prior to 1978, Dr. Wilkinson was Associate Cancer Research Scientist, Roswell Park Memorial Institute, and Associate Professor and Director of Graduate Studies, Program in Epidemiology and Oncology, Roswell Park Graduate Division of the State University of New York at Buffalo.

Dr. Wilkinson has published widely in the areas of public health, health education, and epidemiology. His articles have appeared in the American Journal of Public Health, Public Health Reports, Health Education Monographs, the International Journal of Health Education, Social Science and Medicine, and numerous other professional journals.

Dr. Wilkinson holds a B.A., M.A., and Ph.D. from the State University of New York at Buffalo, and he has completed postdoctoral research at Duke University Medical Center, Durham, North Carolina.